Great Expectation

sightline books
The Iowa Series in Literary Nonfiction
Patricia Hampl & Carl H. Klaus, series editors

Dan Roche
Great Expectation
A Father's Diary

University of Iowa Press, Iowa City

University of Iowa Press, Iowa City 52242
Copyright © 2008 by Dan Roche
www.uiowapress.org
Printed in the United States of America
Text design by Richard Hendel
No part of this book may be reproduced or used
in any form or by any means without permission in
writing from the publisher. All reasonable steps have
been taken to contact copyright holders of material
used in this book. The publisher would be pleased
to make suitable arrangements with any whom it
has not been possible to reach.

The University of Iowa Press is a member of
Green Press Initiative and is committed to
preserving natural resources.
Printed on acid-free paper

These notes were written between
June 2003 and January 2004.

Library of Congress
Cataloging-in-Publication Data
Roche, Daniel, 1958–
   Great expectation: a father's diary / by Dan Roche.
     p.   cm.—(Sightline books: the Iowa series
in literary nonfiction)
   ISBN-13: 978-1-58729-661-1 (cloth)
   ISBN-10: 1-58729-661-6 (cloth)
   1. Roche, Daniel, 1958–   2. Fathers—United
States—Diaries.   3. Fatherhood.   4. Preg-
nancy—Popular works.   5. Infants—Care.
6. Father and infant.   I. Title.
HQ756.R637 2008   2008001896
306.874'2092—dc22

08 09 10 11 12 C 5 4 3 2 1

My thanks to all those who have allowed themselves to be portrayed in these pages, especially Maura and Maeve, and to those who read the manuscript with sharp eyes: Tom Kennedy, Carl Klaus, Mike Streissguth, and Karl Stukenberg.

Great Expectation

JUNE 1

Maura's sprouting a little belly that looks squishy like our daughter's translucent rubber ball with the tiny white frogs in it. When you squeeze the ball one side of it pops up into a bubble, through which the frogs stare creepily at you. I know enough not to squeeze Maura's belly in that way—or describe her belly this way to her—but if I did, the thing that would appear would be just over two inches long and be shaped like a comma. At least that's what it looked like on the ultrasound today.

Maura is eight weeks along and likes her energy. Last night, she was recalling for a friend that she'd never felt better than when she was pregnant the first time around, and that the good feeling has returned.

"Your body's trying to tell you something," he said.

"Well," Maura told him, "it's a good thing I don't have to listen to my body all the time. I'd be in trouble."

Also high on the bonus list at this point, Maura says, is "having cleavage." That and the prospect of eating. And new clothes. Maura's full of smarts and substance—reads philosophy, writes about Milton, is an English professor—but she never discounts the importance and satisfaction of style. On the clothes front, she's relieved because she's just picked up some stretchy tops that are more hip than she was letting herself hope for. One's a reddish tie-dye kind of tunic, and another's a V-neck thing with small flowers, but not overly flowery like the dowdiest maternity clothes are. She also got some Capri pants. During the past couple of years as Maura and I were trying to decide whether we wanted another child, she articulated all kinds of complex reasons for and against. At the moment, though, the best "pro" is that it's an excuse to shop.

If all goes well, this baby will grow to nine or ten pounds, the size of our first child when she was born. They had to do a C-section, and I still remember standing next to the doctor and watching him lift the big baby out like a man hoisting something up over the side of a boat.

We had been keeping the pregnancy a secret up until yesterday, when we told our daughter, Maeve, who is almost five and is a terrible leak. She immediately told a couple of other people. I did want to wait until about twelve weeks, partly because Maura had two miscarriages last year, one at just about this far along, after we had spread the news a week before. Congratulations cards arrived in batches, followed a few days later by sympathy cards. I also thought it'd be nice to dwell for a while longer in a little cocoon, get used to the idea of infancy again, avoid for the time being having to answer the inevitable question of whether I want a boy or a girl. (Answer: Girl. I know something about them now, and we've got all those clothes!)

Anyway, Maura is slender and is showing earlier this time. So we're telling people. The men act surprised, and every woman smiles and says, "I know."

JUNE 2

Maura's sister Jennifer is pregnant too, so babies are growing everywhere. This is also her second. Her first, a boy, is not even two, so she and Andy are getting the creation part out of the way so they can concentrate fully on the rearing part. But Jennifer's not happy about how that strategy is going over in Peoria, where they live. (We live in Syracuse, 700 miles away, unfortunately too far for the pregnant sisters to grow side-by-side.) Jennifer called today pissed because a woman in the grocery store looked at her holding the baby and bulging out under her blouse and sneered, "I would *never* have two so close together."

"What kind of Midwestern graciousness is that?" I asked, even while I was also thinking, Well, isn't having two in diapers really only a step away from having, say, septuplets, at which point you call in the national media so churches and Gerber know to send help?

Jennifer said, "I told her that I'm thirty-eight, we've had trouble, and I'll take what I can get."

"Did it shut her up?"

"She huffed away."

Maura's thirty-nine, so I guess we're taking what we can get, too. I'm forty-five, which worries me even more, because the best working system in my body may be the reproductive one. Everything else is iffy. But at least we'll have an older kid to fetch bottles and entertain herself during the worst of the new-baby chaos—if, in fact, that's what a five-year-old can do.

JUNE 4

I can't say that Maura and I ever seriously considered stopping at one, but it took a long time before we felt ready to go past that. We'd gotten to that point last fall, though after the miscarriages it was a relief to welcome the onset of what people here call a "real" winter, in which it snowed nearly constantly, the temperatures were below normal, and we got a break from the expectation that everything *should* keep on living.

We didn't try for a kid during those cold months. Occasionally, I would broach the subject only because I had a small impatience to give it one more shot, to let the third time seal our fate. At those moments I would find myself thinking possessively of Maura's aging eggs, as if they were little soccer balls she was holding on the sidelines and wouldn't inbound. But she'd be lying in bed and reading something like *Beowulf*—she was teaching a medieval literature course that semester—and thinking about the dark dread of the lurking monsters in that epic poem, and she'd say, "I just need a break."

And then one day in late March, over lunch in a diner, we both seemed to have opened fully to the possibility again. It was a misty and gray day, still destined to snow a couple of more times, but it was *officially* spring, and that brought with it some urgency.

I felt I could go either way, really, on having another kid. It was nice to think about having some time back, now that Maeve was close to going into kindergarten, and I wasn't actually unfulfilled in any parenting sense. But, I said again to Maura as I had many times before, I did want another baby for Maeve's sake. The thought of her growing up without a sibling made me sad, and I thought it would make her so, too, somewhere down the line.

Maura nodded at the wisdom of giving Maeve a brother or sister. She was playing idly with the sugar packets, constructing a little building.

Then she talked about some of her own current motivations. "In those first two years with Maeve," she recalled, "I felt like I was making it up as I went along. I was off-balance. I guess now I want a chance to bring my attention more to taking care of a baby without feeling panicked about it. I want a do-over."

She paused and pushed the sugar packets around slowly with her fingertip, then added, "And of course I want that joy."

JUNE 5

We named Maeve after an old queen of Ireland who had a thing for slicing off the heads of her enemies.

"Well, she was certainly no nun," one Irishman said to Maura and me when we told him about the way we were paying honor to the former ruler. This was just a few weeks ago, when Maura and I were in Ireland celebrating our tenth anniversary. (My parents and Maura's mom had come to Syracuse to babysit our Maeve.) Maura and I hiked to the top of Knocknarea, a modest-sized mountain outside Sligo atop of which Queen Maeve is supposedly buried under a huge pile of rocks. She's very famous locally, in the same way that Daniel Boone is famous in Kentucky. There are restaurants and inns named after her. And it's true that her personality did not approach the saintly. We bought Maeve an illustrated children's version of the legend, and the book tells of Queen Maeve and her husband sitting around bored one evening and comparing who had the most stuff—a typical mid-marriage conversation. When, after several hours of tit-for-tat, Ailill pulled ahead by remembering his wild bull, the queen fumed but decided to get one of her own. War ensued, people were killed, and in the end the bull she got gored Ailill's bull to death and then died of a heart attack. Maybe not the best example of mature behavior, but Maura and I were attracted by the passion and gusto it all represented.

Maeve the Brave, we call our Maeve.

Still, it was good not to have her chattering between us during our week away. A little reprieve before the new one arrives. With such freedom we could have spent all our evenings in pubs drinking Guinness and listening to live music if Maura had been drinking and could stay awake past 8:30. Instead we spent days strolling through small towns in the west, braced and refreshed by the constant wind and frequent rain.

At the Cliffs of Moher we watched crazy people inch to the edge of the stunning dropoff—seven hundred feet straight down to the ocean. We felt dizzy enough well back behind the low rock wall. Just a few hours after we left (we read in the paper the next day) a young woman from Dublin arrived on a tour bus, walked too close to the edge, and was pushed by the wind over the side. A horrific event, but the image stays with me even now in a disturbingly poetic way, ourselves rooted solidly on the rocky and lush island, while at the edge someone is falling helplessly away.

JUNE 6
We met a man in the park this morning whose two kids were playing on the swings while he sat next to us decked out in local sports paraphernalia—a T-shirt commemorating the Syracuse Orangemen's 2003 NCAA basketball championship, a Syracuse University cap, even orange sneakers. When we mentioned to him that Maura was pregnant, he laughed and said, "Ah, you're going from double-team to man-to-man. It's a whole new ballgame."

JUNE 7
The due date is January 8. "Elvis's birthday!" people say. I wouldn't have guessed that so many people know this.

"Oh, they do," my friend Mike pointed out. "January 8 is like Christmas day for the Presleytarians."

At this stage, when there's not much going on with the pregnancy, there's time to think about the significances of birth dates—astrology, if you're into that, or saints' days, if that's your thing. Elvis does not rank up there for me with Queen Maeve as a role model or patron saint, though my mom likes the idea. She's such an Elvis fan that a few years ago we hired an Elvis impersonator for her sixtieth birthday, a guy who pulled his rumbling old white Ford Torino into the driveway, then carried his knee-high amplifier into the backyard and sang "Love Me Tender" with my mom in his arms until she rushed off laughing and came back a few minutes later with a button she'd pinned to her blouse that said "Elvis is Dead, Get a Life." She has a collection of Elvis paraphernalia, both loving and sardonic. The impersonator sang a few more songs, then locked into his final performance-ending karate-like pose—his face scrunched groundward, the mike squeezed tightly at his hunched-over chest, his left arm holding up a fist, his legs poised as if he might be thinking of crouching down to pick something up. Then he relaxed, stood up straight, unplugged his amp, and hung around for a piece of birthday cake. After he left a few minutes later, my dad came back from around front to announce that Elvis's car had leaked oil onto his concrete driveway.

Having people shout excitedly that our baby is due to share a birthday with Elvis feels a little bit like something unwelcome is leaking into the scenario. Maybe I should go with it, though, be as excited as my brother was when his son was born not on December 6, my birthday, but on December 7, Larry Bird's birthday.

JUNE 10

I can only think that it's displaced fear over the vulnerability of that little comma-shaped frog in her belly that is causing Maura to do what she is doing with Perry, our twelve-year-old cat, who got an abscess on his cheek last week. It's his second this year. Most likely he scratched himself, since he's not one of those cats that prowls the neighborhood all night and drags himself home at dawn with half an ear missing and his fur matted with blood. He's big and self-confident and has more class. He pretty much stays in the backyard, and if another cat encroaches upon that territory, Perry makes a burly feint, and the intruder slinks away.

But Perry is FIV-positive, the feline equivalent to HIV. Not that it ever caused him much problem. The worst sickness I've ever seen him have was a disgusting cold during which he kept sneezing black snot all over the window screens. Now, though, the abscesses have reminded Maura that Perry skates on thin ice. It's a return to the first years after we found out about the FIV, when Maura cooked him daily meals of vegetables and raw chicken. That gravy train eventually stopped, but it always stands as a sign of how far Maura will go for this cat's sake.

Now, Maura says, Perry can't go out. She claims this is to keep him alive longer, but he's been an outdoor cat for so long that it's hard to imagine he'd choose to live any other kind of life. For days after his sentence was handed down, he charged toward the door whenever anyone went in that direction, but then he soon began lying on his side and following you to the door with only his eyes. Then sometimes he didn't even open his eyes.

Maura's got Maeve trained in this madness, and now whenever someone opens the back door and Perry makes a slow move for freedom, she begins yelling, "No, Perry! No! Stay there, Perry!" It's a really loud voice, and it breaks all sense of peacefulness that having a mellow cat ought to bring. It's even worse because when Perry does squeeze past the door, he goes to the bottom of the five steps and lies down on the warm bricks of the patio. The cat has never run more than six feet in his life. (When we had a party a few months ago, Perry sat on the kitchen table while people were coming in to get beers from the fridge. One person looked long and hard at him, holding the refrigerator door wide open, and then asked, "Is that a real cat?")

"Well, you've broken his spirit," I told Maura.

She insists he's perfectly happy indoors.

I whisper to Perry that once the baby comes, he'll be liberated again. It fails to perk him up.

JUNE 12

I've been trying to remember the details of when Maura was pregnant with Maeve, just in case anything might come in handy this time around. But it all seems so long ago, as indistinct as if I'm looking at it all through a shower curtain.

Maura and I complement each other because her *short*-term memory stinks. And it's worse when she's pregnant. She reminded me this morning of how she was always forgetting her house keys the last time around. We were living in Arkansas at the time, and usually, after the door locked behind her, Maura would sit on the front porch and look longingly through the front window at a stack of magazines on the coffee table, wishing she'd at least remembered to carry one with her. An hour or two later I'd get home and let her in. One day she simply got a crowbar out of the garage and smashed out a window in the back door, then reached in and unlocked it. Our eighty-five-year-old neighbor Mary Lou moseyed over and asked politely if everything was all right. Mary Lou was a wonderful old Arkansas woman who, when Maura first told her she was pregnant, had replied, "I suspicioned as much." She was always suspicioning things, often with good cause, such as looking out her window to see Maura come out of the garage with a crowbar and then hearing glass tinkling against the tile floor. We should have given Mary Lou an extra key during those months, but Maura kept forgetting to do it.

Maura's first pregnancy was only half a decade ago, but I might as well be trying to remember what happened when my mother was pregnant with me. I suspicion that something of what went on back then I could put to use this time, but it's not coming to me.

JUNE 16

Maura has canned her doctor, who was approaching the pregnancy like a NASCAR pit boss, measuring blood levels every week, checking eye pressure and electrolyte concentrations and who knows what else. At eleven weeks it seems early to be checking for dilation, but this doctor stopped just short of that. All this because of the two miscarriages last year.

Maura wants someone less medical, which sounds like wanting a barber who's not that much into hair. Really what she wants, as she told me, is a doctor who will allow her *not* to think or worry about her body and the baby every waking moment of the day. "I don't want more control," she explained, "I want less. Less information, fewer choices, greater simplicity."

Not ignorance, she says, but the slow and quiet naturalness that can seem almost like a privilege in these days of high technology. Enough of the lurking monsters.

It is not simplicity, however, that Maura has been getting so far from Doctor #2 — a woman whose greatest virtue, it turns out, is that her office is right down the street. Location might be the prime consideration in choosing, say, a muffler shop, but it's not a terrible thing to have to drive across town for the right physician.

This doctor's flaw is that she has a specialty: pregnant women with Marfan's Syndrome — a disconcerting condition in which your connective tissue is weak, leading to things like your heart coming apart if you put too much stress on it, such as if you, say, push hard during labor. Marfan's sufferers are characteristically tall and thin, as Maura is.

"Are you sure you don't have Marfan's?" this doctor asked Maura almost immediately. She might as well have said, "Do you want your husband to raise the child alone or would you prefer he get remarried right away?"

Actually, Marfan's women can have babies, Maura reported to me — she spent most of last night on the Internet reading about it — but the risks are high, right up there in the category with a nineteenth-century frontier woman having triplets in a log cabin or a twenty-first-century woman trying to begin motherhood at fifty. Maura didn't look confident about the odds. In fact, she looked as if she were waiting for her body to shred apart at any minute, like pulled pork.

I tried to put things in perspective. "*No* one's ever mentioned Marfan's before," I said. "Does that make sense?"

"It's not always obvious," she argued. She'd found pictures of women on Marfan's web sites who didn't look like Abe Lincoln, whom some people consider the Marfan's poster child.

She's sitting downstairs right now, calling up every woman in town she knows who's had a kid. I think she's approaching this medical threat in exactly the right way, by finding a new doctor with a better prognosis.

JUNE 18

Doctor #3 wears cowboy boots, like a large-animal vet. He also seems thoroughly practical and sensible. "You don't have Marfan's," he told Maura. "You've got no signs at all."

He did an ultrasound, showing us the heart beating, a tiny blip in the gray screen, like a helicopter hovering on radar.

"What you've got is a baby," he said, seeming genuinely thrilled.

JUNE 19

Even with the new doctor's confidence and heartiness, there are vague and unlikely things to worry about. We're reminded of one every time we glance at the kitchen counter, where for months there has been sitting a chromosome map of Maura's older sister, Sheila. It's a private thing to leave out, like a bad report card, but probably no one who's seen it has been able to decipher it. It looks vaguely genetic, but it also looks like a piece of paper that was left too close to the stove and had drops of tomato soup splashed on it.

Maura got the map from her mom, who had to dig it out of a box. Some scientists made it when Sheila was one or two, as proof that she had Down syndrome.

Sheila is now forty, and as far as I know she's unaware that we have this little window into her being. Whenever I've seen her recently, I've felt a moment of awkwardness, because even though she is smart and witty and fully capable of engaging in important conversations, it would seem rude to say to her, as I want to, "So, I was looking at your chromosomal map the other day."

Maura wanted the map because she has a low-level worry about this baby being retarded. The fear is working its way into Maura's dreams, and even into her half-waking moments. She told me this morning that there was a voice talking to her last night before she went to sleep, a voice that said that this was going to be an "exceptional" child.

"It didn't say what it meant by that," Maura explained, "except that it added that everything was going to be okay."

I asked whether it was a male or female voice.

"It was more like a written voice than a spoken voice," Maura said. "A voice from the page. It even spelled out the word: *exceptional*."

Maura also has a cousin who is so profoundly retarded that she's never walked or talked. Claire is Sheila's age.

"It's just coincidence," Maura's mom says whenever Maura presses her for theories on why these two retardations occurred in tandem. These are the only two cases in any generation of her family, as far as anyone knows. When Maura brings it up with doctors, they shrug and tell her that Down's is not hereditary. Still, she holds on to the map, as a talisman, a paper worry-stone.

JUNE 20

The upcoming baby—until enough information or imagination comes along that changes things—has officially been named the Very Young Elvis.

This per our friend Bonnie, who is visiting with her husband, Mike, and their kids, Aiden and Esmé. It's been like *Cheaper by the Dozen* around here these last few days, because Bonnie and Mike used to live down the street (before Mike joined the Foreign Service and they all moved to Bulgaria—a scenario out of some inexplicable 1940s film noir), and so all of the kids' old friends have been coming over to hang out with them too. One side of the living room has been covered in platoons of small plastic army soldiers in the midst of battle—courtesy of Aiden and his buddies. The other side of the room is covered with a dozen or two Polly Pockets and enough clothes and accessories for the Pollys *and* the army—courtesy of Esmé and Maeve.

The noise is absolutely constant and high, like a factory or a Harley convention. The Very Young Elvis must be hearing all this and either wanting to peer out for a look or trying to reach his little arm buds up to cover his ears.

JUNE 22

Bonnie has been doing some work over in Bulgaria with orphanages, and the stories she brought back are the kind that make you feel about as crummy as you can for not immediately flying there and adopting any abandoned kid with so much as a runny nose. In fact, *every* abandoned kid—most of whose real problems are much worse. Kids left alone on mattresses that reek from urine. Orphanages so undersupplied that there are not enough spoons for every child to eat at the same time. It's hard to hear.

"I can give you a contact," Bonnie said. "I can get you a kid for, like, four or five thousand."

She couldn't have expected an answer. The only *sane* thing would've been to say yes.

It made me wish, for only the briefest of moments, that Maura and I were one of those born-again Christian couples with the unrelenting smiles and the double-knit slacks, the ones who get written up every so often in the paper. There's always a picture of them in a shiny kitchen with ten kids.

JUNE 26

Maura's into the second trimester now, and I *have* remembered one important thing about this phase from her first pregnancy. There were a couple of months there when her hormones had kicked into such high gear that, like an eighteen-year-old guy, she could barely keep her mind off sex. I reminded Maura of the experience the other day, and she seemed to have her own nostalgic fascination for it, as if it had been like a semester abroad. "These ideas would pop into my head," she recalled, "and I'd think, 'Hmm, I wonder what *that* would be like.'"

Too early to tell right now whether history will repeat itself. It helped last time, I have to say, that we didn't have any kids to intrude upon those unbidden fantasies.

JUNE 28

We're dogsitting. It's Calvin, Maura's mom's big collie. He's ancient—thirteen years old—and we're hoping he doesn't die on our watch. Still, Gail—in a voice that was more upbeat and matter-of-fact than I thought she might want to use around the dog himself—gave us the go-ahead to "do whatever you need to" while she's away.

Calvin has a bad spine. When he wants to lie down it takes him fifteen or twenty minutes of pacing in circles, his back feet splayed out, before he gets the courage to let himself fall through the pain to the floor—like a person wanting to swallow big pills and tossing his head back six or eight times before they get over the hump and go down the throat. When he wants to get back up, he grimaces and his back paws strain for traction, like someone trying to pull a car out of a snowy ditch.

Since he can't bend very well anymore, and since he also can't go in reverse, he'll often get his nose into a tight corner to sniff something and I'll have to lift him up and turn him around. His turning radius is about twenty feet. We have a narrow passageway in the kitchen between the refrigerator and a cabinet, and Calvin often ends up standing sideways across it, so that all traffic comes to a complete halt until he inches his way out of his jam. It's like having our own private lock-and-dam system.

JUNE 30

I've been volunteering for the past year as an EMT, mostly as a way to make up for not going to med school twenty years ago. (I became an engineer instead, and then chucked that after a while to become an

English professor.) Once a week I go sit at the fire station and wait for the alarm to go off, and when we go on a call I'm the rookie who takes vital signs, gets patient histories, and occasionally helps someone administer an albuterol treatment for emphysema. There's always also a paramedic on hand to do the gory needle-sticking, intubations, and defibrillating.

Last night my job was to hold a big piece of gauze bandage against a lady's scalp. She'd fallen on her back porch. While I was waiting for the bleeding to stop, the woman's neighbor walked across the yard, drink in hand, and started announcing, "These guys are the best! These guys are heroes!" In his loopy state, he kept pointing to me as exactly what he was talking about.

I let him rant.

Being an EMT seems pleasant and hobby-like to me, but that's probably because I haven't yet been to any car wrecks or shootings. So far, it's like being in a pregnancy but before any kids are actually born. Still, the words of my teacher from last year are fresh. He liked to scare us into the seriousness of what we'd undertaken.

"You get infected by a patient who has nontreatable tuberculosis," he would say, "you're gonna die." Or: "You put a patient with congestive heart failure in the supine position, he's gonna die." Those last three words were always flat and blunt, like something from a video game. He drew out "die" ever so slightly, and let his voice drop a notch, then left the word hanging in the air.

JULY 1

In the paper this morning was an article about severely disabled children. I'd read the paper first and momentarily considered slipping that section into the recycling bin before Maura saw it. But she did see it — a big picture of a woman tending to her fifteen-year-old multiply handicapped boy.

"We need to talk about testing," Maura said.

Neither of us has been inclined to test. After a talking-out, I figured, testing would ultimately seem to her just the kind of thing she was getting away from by dropping her first OB. Still, this quick combination of first Maura's dream and then this article — a one-two punch coming at a time when we're feeling a little wary—made the talking-out, at least, seem worthwhile.

Maura felt her way into it, articulating some of her fears about what might befall this baby, and what our lives might be like as a consequence. I listened and agreed with the worst of the projections—or at least agreed that they'd be difficult beyond imagining. But the problem for me was that everything was beyond imagining, even with the picture from the paper there in front of me. I can hardly put myself in the place of those whose luck has been worse than I assume mine will be. That sounds like a terrible lack of empathy. And maybe it is, since empathy springs from imagination. I don't like to think of myself as lacking empathy, but the truth is that when it comes to predicting troubles I might encounter down the road, my vision is about as reliable as the average person's—which is to say that it's as if I'm in a steam room, barely able to make out the features of the person next to me.

And yet I hang onto this youthful optimism, which at moments seems to me the only sane way to become a parent again at my age. But of course it's all counterbalanced by the depressing fears of death that color my mid-forties: not just mine but those of Maura and Maeve. I'm constantly surprised to see them springing around me happily alive and healthy. Beyond our own family, of course, there is the state of the world itself, with color-coded threat warnings for terrorism, with bombs and guns that are generally far from my little village but seemingly as likely to go off here as they are in Oklahoma City or on the train we occasionally ride down to New York City. Last night I was reading Kathleen Norris's book *Dakota*, and I stopped when she quoted this line from Benedict: "Day to day remind yourself that you are going to die." I understand that this approach is supposed to make one live a fuller life. It's a belief both harder and more comforting to hold onto as one gets older.

So I'm torn on how to think about the dangers of this pregnancy, though I'm sure I'll end up doing what has been both my strength and my weakness all my life: to take things as they come. It's a quality that would make me a lousy doctor, an inept politician. But I keep falling back on that strategy because what's come so far in my life has been bearable and even good—no deaths closer than a grandparent, no illnesses of lasting or debilitating nature, a divorce that was deeply painful but better than staying married.

Maura spoke on, recalling that we didn't test when she was pregnant with Maeve, even though she was thirty-four — right on the cusp of "advanced maternal age," when a pregnant woman is generally encouraged to walk gingerly and expect the worst.

Finally I asked, "What would you do if the tests did show something?"

She pursed her lips. This was the real question, the one that might give this potential information some practical value. So much of what we can learn has none of that — such as finding out, as we did about Maura's second miscarriage after her OB insisted on sending a tissue sample to the genetics lab, that the fetus was "Trisome 16. Incompatible with life." I've tried many times to find some use in that fact, but it remains only a lump of curiosity. And what do I do with the knowledge — also the result of that analysis — that the baby would've been a girl? Where does one store that? Joan Didion famously said that we tell ourselves stories in order to live. If the facts never rise to a story, is their burden too heavy?

"From what I've read," Maura said, "even with an amnio, they can't say with all that much accuracy what might happen. I don't think I'd do anything."

I pursed my own lips and turned my hands palms up, to indicate that we'd reasoned ourselves into an answer. It's not a perfect answer, and I suspect we'll both continue to fear that we're burying our heads in the sand, turning blind eyes to knowledge. This is not the way that two college professors usually approach the world, trained as we are, to hear our students say it, to overanalyze everything. But you choose your burdens, choose your worries.

JULY 5

We feel comfortable with the new OB, as if we've been rewarded with something exactly right after a couple of missteps. He has the right combination of relaxation and focus, joking around while at the same time inhabiting the small exam room with professionalism and ease, and he clearly knows his boundaries, acknowledging the obvious fact that Maura and I are hardly naïve teenagers who've gotten themselves into a bind. I think I may even be older than he is. When we asked him about testing, he said he'd set it up for us if we wanted, but that he'd be perfectly comfortable with skipping that altogether. His great talent is in quickly dismissing our inessential fears.

It was a surprise, then, when we had our friend Tom over for dinner and told him that we were using this doctor. At the mention of his name Tom nodded knowingly, the muscles on his face tight.

"What?" I asked.

Tom is in his late forties and has a charmingly pessimistic view of certain things. For years he worked in banking, handling bankruptcies, and last year he quit his job to go to law school and become a bankruptcy attorney. I mentioned to him the first time I met him that I was toying with the idea of opening a bookstore in the little village where we live.

"It won't work," he had announced with quick certitude that took me aback but also impressed me. "You can't compete with the chains." He then laid out for me exactly how he saw my finances plunging as soon as I stepped into the idealistic world of the independent bookstore, exactly how sorry was my imagination of everything that would go wrong. He'd seen it happen over and over.

I didn't hold the pessimism against him. Actually, I felt refreshed by the depth of his convictions, even if for a while I continued to think he was absolutely wrong. Faced with the stories of the failures of other people to accomplish the very thing I have in mind, I usually first wonder what those stories have to do with me. I'm a temporary optimist, but I like pessimists because I usually come around to their dark views after I spend enough time enjoying my own rosy visions.

"He's an anti-abortionist who, if it came to it, would choose the baby's life over the mother's life like that," Tom said. He snapped his fingers. "You'd better ask him about this," he said, looking at me. He moved his head back and forth slowly and let his eyelids droop behind his wire-rim glasses — a look he clearly perfected through years of talking to people who've lost all their money. It's not a sympathetic look, exactly, but there's an odd sense of reassurance to it, something that can make people shake their own heads and mutter, "I know, I know." I think he has a great future as a lawyer. He lifted his beer bottle and let it swing between index and middle fingers.

"Well," I said, "this explains the cowboy boots."

Maura let out a little puff of air and rolled her eyes. She doesn't have a lot of patience whenever someone questions a decision she's already made. I've found this out repeatedly over the years and have gradually shared with her less and less information that I know would be beneficial. For instance, when she's driving, I mostly keep my mouth shut about shortcuts that she seems to have no conception of or interest in. Amazingly, in the car and in all other ways, she usually turns out okay, as if she'd really known all along what was best for her. I'm constantly surprised.

But Tom's information was different. This was life and death.

"He does refer to the fetus as 'baby,' you know," I added, "the way a right-winger would."

"So does Maeve," Maura pointed out. "So do we."

"This doesn't worry you?" I asked. I wasn't sure whether I wanted to be worried about it, but Tom's seriousness had me a little rattled. What did he know?

"Look," Maura said, "I don't need a doctor who's going to go to pro-choice rallies with me. What I want is someone who will take care of me in this pregnancy the way I want to be taken care of, and he's doing that. He's excellent."

"Oh, I've no doubt he knows his stuff," Tom said, solid in the face of Maura's decisiveness. "It's just this one thing." He shrugged and looked at me again. "It seems like an important thing to me, but. . . ."

JULY 8
Our OB seemed less likable when we went to visit him next, three days after Tom had recharacterized him for us. He was a little pudgier, a little less charismatic, a little more dangerous looking. It may have had something to do with the fact that we had to wait more than an hour before seeing him, and the fact that he'd delivered a baby at 2:00 that morning and hadn't been back to bed since. But who knew?

It didn't help his case when he couldn't find the fetus's heartbeat. He was pressing a small microphone-like gadget against Maura's lower belly, but all that came out of the transistor-radio-sized speaker attached to it was static.

"Is that the baby's heartbeat?" Maeve asked, looking up from her coloring book in the corner.

"No," I told her, trying to sound patient. "That's just static, dear."

The doctor was staring at Maura's belly as he searched.

"This is the most difficult time to find them," he said. "There's a lot of fluid relative to baby."

After two minutes he gave up.

"We could do an ultrasound," he immediately offered. "It's completely up to you, but if you'd sleep better tonight, I'll go get the ultrasound machine."

"Yes," I said.

And there was the baby, all fifty millimeters of it, with a head and a tookus and a blip-blip of a heartbeat. I held Maeve up so she could see the screen, and the doctor printed several copies of the image for us to take home.

Maeve and I took them out to the sidewalk, and I studied them while Maeve ate the lollipop she got from the nurse's desk and Maura hung around inside to ask the doctor a few more questions: about diet, about weight gain, about rates of incidence of pre-eclampsia for older pregnant women. I didn't remind her to ask the doctor about the abortion thing, but when she came out a few minutes later, I looked at her expectantly. She shook her head in the tiniest, annoyed way.

"If you want to ask him, go ahead," she said. "It's not an issue for me. I'm not bringing it up."

JULY 9

Last night I was out for a walk and stopped to talk to my neighbor Tim, who was in his garage building an airplane—a replica of a 1929 single-seater that he says he'll fly when it's done. Tim's a good guy, and a brilliant engineer, and he told me in fascinating detail how chocolate is manufactured, including how they have to temper it to get it to flow through the four-inch pipes throughout the factory. Stuff he learned from having to do a survey of a chocolate factory a few months ago. At another point, he said, "I've always wondered how they roll the tops of paper cups," and then he explained it to me, and then added with a self-deprecatory shrug, "I have weird obsessions." I smiled and nodded and tried to use words like "compression" and "extraction" and "temper" in sentences of my own. Kept trying to come up with something new to say that would be *just as good* as what he was saying.

It was a stupid sense of competition, and I don't think Tim even noticed it, but I left his garage feeling foolish. And thinking, in an anxious sort of way, that the idea of having a boy scares me more than, say, the idea of having a pit bull. Well, maybe about the same.

Who knows where this self-consciousness with being around other men—or boys, for that matter—comes from? It's lifelong, I know that, and I suppose I should be more interested in understanding it so that I could cure it. But, man, that's work that doesn't appeal to me. And it doesn't even seem that urgent, because most of the time I can play the guy role pretty well, mixing it up in pickup basketball games, playing racquetball twice a week with my friend Mike, changing the wheel bearings on my car, almost always renting war movies when I go to the video store. Volunteering as an EMT. Altruism, you know. Help out the community. But what I really wanted was to go to the local fire station for a few hours each week and get my undiluted but limited dose of conversation about motorcycles and fire and women and college football and knee injuries. Jab around a little. It's energizing and exhausting, like any stimulant is.

The other day I was playing Chutes and Ladders with Maeve, and, as she always does, she put the fix in so that we both won the same number of times. This is "fair."

And when I'm sitting across the table from her rather than from any male, it does seem harmlessly and even productively fair. Not that I've been able to carry over any of that feeling into some of my talks with guys. In the worst of those, I still end up sounding like the White House spokesman for a really stupid president: self-protective and full of rationalizations.

I don't know. Maybe I'm in this phase right now because I'm heading inexorably into more domesticity, with the upcoming baby care and all that. It's going to cut me off for a year, maybe two, from my male friends, just as it did when Maeve was a baby and nearly all of my free time was with her.

Whatever it is, I almost never feel competitive with a woman, no matter how smart she is.

I'm not sure I'm up for the competition of having a son.

JULY 10

Maura reminds me that when we found out Maeve was going to be a girl, I turned to her and asked, "What do you *do* with a girl?" I'd forgotten. But now, raising a girl seems like the only thing I can know about kids.

JULY 12

I've been going through the name books and making lists. I'm trying very hard to be open, to see the art and energy in all names, to listen closely for the mellifluousness, for whatever speaks to me. There's a list sitting now on the kitchen table. The left column, of girls' names, is the length of the page. In the right column, there are three boys' names, one of which I knew even as I wrote it down I didn't like. I put it there as filler.

Stylistically speaking, having (or being, for that matter) a boy is a life of limitations. There are only a few names of interest. You go into the boys' section of a clothes store and there's about as much selection as in a janitorial supply shop. When you really don't need a kid who can hold up one side of the tractor while you change the flat tire, it's really beyond me why anyone would want a boy.

They do, of course — or at least they act that way, though I suspect what's really at work is something no one admits to, except people like Maura's friend, who told her recently, "I love all my children equally, but there's something special about the bond between a mother and a son. Maybe it's because we feel sorry for them."

I feel sorry for boys. Not, of course, for their privileges, their higher average annual salaries, their historical entitlements as brokers of power, their luck at being able to pee standing up. It boils down to my own male guilt in the ruination of the world. That's all.

JULY 14

We spent the last few days in New Jersey with a boy. He's four. As with most little boys, I didn't know what to do with him. He knew what he wanted from me, though, which was to play catch. And more catch. I played, until it got tiring because he couldn't get the ball all the way to me, and then I told him to go into the nearby woods and make a fort. Off he trotted, and I sat back down on the park bench like any old person ought to do.

This boy's voice is deep and husky, as if it's already changed. And he doesn't smile much, just has this serious look like you're supposed to know what he's thinking. If *I'm* noticing that already, just wait until he's eighteen and gives that look to a girlfriend.

But he's a good kid, and with a little coaching from his parents he probably won't grow up to be one of those Jersey thugs who wears black concert T-shirts with the sleeves cut off.

And now this week we've got a boy right here in the house. It's my nephew Eamon, who brought along his mom and dad, Jennifer and Andy, as roadies. Eamon is fifteen months old, and I haven't decided yet whether I'm going to try to be friends with him, or whether I'll wait for his sister to be born in October. (Jennifer is out to *here*.) So far, he hasn't caused any trouble or done much that a girl probably wouldn't do, but he's only been here twenty-four hours.

Maeve has the same suspicion of a boy's long-term worth. Last night, she had been playing with Eamon for a couple of hours, the two of them laughing and having all kinds of fun. Then someone who obviously doesn't understand the depth of her convictions asked her whether she'd like to have a baby brother. She didn't hesitate, didn't get thrown off focus because of one good date—a promising sign for later years. "I want a sister," she said firmly.

Andy has what seems like a modest but realistic goal concerning his son. "I don't care if he's not smart," he says, "as long as he's not an ass."

JULY 15

In the park this morning, Jennifer asked me whether I was rooting for a girl or a boy. We were watching Eamon play with the buckles on his stroller, trying to decipher the code. I didn't want to diss boys in the midst of that cute-son scene, but I told her anyway that any boy I could conjure up in my imagination was running a very distant second to any imagined girl, who was based heavily on Maeve.

Even as I said it, though, I didn't feel as certain in my preference as I had even a few days ago. "It's more the *idea* of boys that I don't want than it is any particular boy," I tried to explain. Eamon's another one of those kids who looks like he may avoid the worst of his gender's faults. Then again, he's not even grunting yet. Instead, he does these cute little birdcall noises, and those make it impossible to judge him with any accuracy.

"You know," I said, "I've *been* a boy. Lots of it was okay, but do I really want to go through it again? Raising a girl is new. It's interesting."

"But maybe raising a boy differently from the way you were raised would be fresh, too?" Jennifer suggested.

The truth is, at my age, I wonder what energy I'll have to get through another kid at all, much less come up with innovative ways to make up for the errors of every previous generation of parents. Still, if energy has to be expended, I'd rather expend it teaching a human how to be strong and independent than teaching one how to ease up on the throttle and not mow down pedestrians.

I see how I'm plugging boys and girls into my own narrow tracks, ignoring the idea that what most males really need is to be taught *different* ways to be strong and independent. Maybe having a boy would be good if only to derail that particular train.

Today at Maeve's swim lesson I sat next to a woman who was burying her face in her hands out of embarrassment over her son's behavior. Whenever the teacher would tell the kids to do ten hops, he'd do thirty, counting out really loudly. Somehow he got put in charge of Red Light, Green Light, and he yelled out the directions without a pause between: "Red light green light red light green light red light. . . ." The teacher said gently, "Could you say them a little slower?" Pretty soon, the teacher and the other kids began ignoring him.

"Christopher, you have got to settle down," the mom would hiss whenever the boy would look at her and she could bear to look at him.

Afterward, she gave him a little lecture. "Every time someone gives you directions, you have to change them to your own fancy," she said. "And it's ex*haus*ting."

JULY 16

I so clearly remember how weak I was with love for Maeve in her first years. I'd be trying to type a letter to her, something for the collection I plan to give her at fifteen to help her break through the teenage funk and see her parents as something other than wrinkled prison wardens, and my arms would be floppy with emotion. I still often get butterflies, feel the weakness in my arms. It's like when I try to put her socks and shoes on her and she's thinking about something else and not bothering at all to point her toes or hold her foot steady. "You've got floppy foot," I tell her. Now it's a big joke, and she likes to get floppy legs and arms, too.

No matter what the baby is, I'm preparing myself for a new immersion in floppiness. I only wonder how it will possibly match what I felt with Maeve. I worry it'll feel mechanical—even dangerous, a threat to the love I feel for both Maeve and Maura. Where is the new love going to come from?

For the moment, I try only to concentrate on the promise I made to myself when Maeve was born: that I would always tell her I love her. Not simply love her, but actually tell her often. As soon as she was born, I said it to her all the time, trying not only to instill the confidence of being loved deep into her body, but also to instill the habit into myself of speaking the words.

JULY 18

For the last two days I've been weighed down by a cloud of sadness. Our old friend Patricia, in Iowa, has died. She'd been battling leukemia for the past six months, a disease that had struck her out of the blue. She fought incredibly hard, even having a bone-marrow transplant two months ago, but the week before last she had a stroke and then died the next day. I only found out about it when Patricia's sister, Rita, who lives here in Syracuse, called to tell us.

Patricia was a single mom, raising her daughter Ria ever since Patricia got divorced when Ria was still very young. Patricia didn't make it easy on herself as a parent, deciding when she was about forty that she wanted to be a writer. Ria was only in fourth grade, and Patricia packed all their stuff in a car and moved them from Florida to Iowa City. The first class she took was one I was teaching, and Ria sat at a desk in the corner drawing pictures. Over the next dozen or so years, Patricia kept going on and on, taking classes, getting her B.A., then her M.F.A., then into a Ph.D. program—along the line she'd gotten interested in educational theories. She was trying to finish her dissertation when she got sick. She scraped by for all those years, living off student loans, teaching-assistantship stipends, and food from her garden. Patricia didn't seem to have any qualms about getting the maximum in student loans every single year—amazingly, the government kept giving them to her—and she couldn't have had any expectation of ever being able to pay them off. I admired her cavalier attitude toward financing, but such debt would have driven me straight to a cubicle from which I'd interrupt people's dinners trying to sell them aluminum siding. Still, I think Patricia did whatever she had to for Ria, keeping the both of them from having to live week-to-week in a crummy motel room with a kitchenette. In fact, they lived in a pleasant yellow house around the corner from us, the two of them seeming to be very happy with each other. Ria helped by being a wonderful and smart kid, full of patience for her mom's undoubtedly difficult decisions, an honors student, a swimmer, a catsitter for us. She graduated from college this spring, and she was back home with her mom at the end.

During her treatment, Patricia wrote the most amazing email dispatches, which she sent out to a bunch of her friends and family. They were heart-wrenching tales of her struggles, usually written from her hospital bed in the middle of the night. She sacrificed more than almost anybody I know in order to be a writer — while simultaneously trying to be a responsible parent — and it's either ironic or fitting that the best writing she ever did came in those dispatches, when she was often so out of it that she could barely focus enough to string words together, much less type them.

My phone conversation with her sister Rita was filled with lots of the typical stiff-upper-lipness that goes along with trying to feel relieved that the suffering is over. But Rita said that quite frequently she just feels this incredible sadness envelop her, and then she has to shake it off. Or pray. Before we hung up, I got to tell her that Maura was pregnant, and she was so thrilled, so enthusiastically happy. It felt like I'd been able to offer a gift during her grieving.

JULY 19

It's been three days since I found out about Patricia's death, and I have hardly been able to write. My entire body feels as if it's soaked up its weight in water. I don't know how to wring myself out. I tried to run yesterday, but gave up after two blocks and came home and ate Nilla Wafers. All I really want to do is sleep.

When I did get to sleep last night, I dreamt about football — a game I haven't liked much since I was twelve. In the dream, the game was going to be violent, and it was clear to me beforehand that I was going to have to throw myself in front of the churning and bony legs of the opposing halfback. I don't think the dream got that far, but I still remember those legs clearly, with the dark hair just below the shiny kneecap. I told Maura that it had to be a dream about having a boy.

We go in next Monday for the fifteen-week checkup. Maybe we'll be able to find out just what's growing in there.

JULY 20

At dinner last night, I asked Maura, "So, what do you think? Boy or girl?"

She didn't jump into the trap. She's tactful on these things. But after a minute she said, slowly and as if she were a little embarrassed, "I have to admit that I'm having a slight preference for a boy."

"No," I said.

She screwed up her face apologetically.

"It's not a *strong* preference, but. . . . And to tell you the truth, I don't know where it's coming from."

"Was it Willie?" I asked.

"He's awful cute," she admitted.

I breathed out in mock exasperation, like I do whenever she sees a magazine cover of Kevin Bacon and has the same reaction. But in Willie's presence I'd also constantly felt myself crumbling like a twelve-year-old girl, so I didn't have much room to talk. Willie is the three-year-old son of our friends Mike and Leslie, and we had dinner at their house the other night. The kid's as adorable as one of those major league bat boys, like Cal Ripken Jr.'s son or something, except more real. I could barely keep from picking him up and cuddling him against my shoulder when he began singing "I went down down down in that burning wing of fiwe." His dad's a big Johnny Cash fan.

"You know the difference between Willie and the boys you fear, don't you?" Maura asked. "I mean the ones who can speak rather than act everything out physically?"

"What?"

"Older sisters."

This was a factor I hadn't considered. Willie's world is colored completely by Emily, seven, and Cate, five, to whom he is constantly yelling, "Wait for me!" He clearly lets some elements of their civilization rub off on him. Finally, a small, open window in the tall, dark wall of boydom I've been imagining.

Maeve was taken by Willie's cuteness, too. She was swinging him around the living room in a tortured kind of dance as she sang "Careless Love," a bluegrass song Maura has taught her as a lullaby, even though it's about a young woman who gets pregnant out of wedlock. I'm thinking that her own loyalty to the idea of a sister may be softening.

JULY 21

Then at swimming lessons this morning, Christopher was his usual self.

"He's got 'dork' written right in the middle of his forehead," Maura said with some sympathy, though I think that will be one of the kinder things he'll be called in the next ten years.

"God help us if we get one like that," I said.

"You don't get other people's children, dear," Maura said wisely.

Maeve's friend Anya was over for playtime today. Anya is five, and had something to teach Maeve. She recited it over lunch:

Girls go to college, get more knowledge.
Boys go to Jupiter, get more stupider.

Then she added, from experience it seemed, "If you have a brother, don't say that in front of him, or else he'll pound you like a bug."

A check-up today. What we learned, as the OB put it, was that we've got "quite a critter in there." He'd found the heartbeat with his little microphone, and it was going clippity-clop, clippity-clop. "You might want to take the kid right to Vernon Downs," he said, meaning the nearest racetrack. "You can name him Lucky."

That was it: confirmation of a living fetus, the sex to remain a mystery. The doctor seemed pleased to stop there and turn his attention to us.

"Got any worries?" he asked.

Maura told him she'd like to be putting on more weight (only two pounds in the last month), but the doctor waved his hand and declared her perfect.

"The only thing I worry about is having a boy," I said.

"Ah, boys are easier," he said jovially and immediately, as everyone seems to say.

I argued. "Nothing could be easier than raising Maeve," I told him. "She's about as much trouble as a houseplant."

He smiled but leaned back against the linoleum counter and settled in to tell me everything I didn't know.

"You see, with girls," he began, "you've got to talk to them and figure them out. Everything's complicated. Boys, they play. If they put their hand through a plate-glass window, they hold it up and say, 'Cool.'"

I admit that Maeve *has* been "sensitive" about some things. There was the time when she was getting close to being potty-trained and messed a pair of panties that had Cinderella on them. Maura was washing them out in the toilet and flushed, only to have the panties be sucked out of her fingers and down the tube. Maeve saw the whole thing and was inconsolable. For forty-five minutes she bawled — still a personal best. Maura comforted her on the sofa, but couldn't make any inroads. Finally, through the exhausted sputtering of her shaking lips, Maeve was able to explain why she was so upset. "Now Snow White won't have a friend!" she cried, and then began bawling again.

She wasn't traumatized for herself. She was empathizing with another pair of underwear.

I'll take that kind of "complication" over a boy's wish to flush *more* underwear down the toilet.

JULY 22

Maeve's aware of her sensitivity, as we discovered when we heard her responding to a neighbor boy who was calling her a crybaby.

"I'm sensitive," Maeve told him.

"You don't even know what that means," he said.

"Yes, I do," she explained slowly, as if the concept would be hard for him to grasp. "It means that when I get hurt, it hurts more."

JULY 24

Maeve's been waking up in the middle of the night two or three times a week lately, padding softly into our room. If she walks around to my side of the bed, she stands over me staring until I wake up. If she goes to Maura's side, she puts her fingers gently on Maura's face, which unfailingly freaks Maura out. She's never ready for it.

Last night, Maeve must've come in about 3:00, though I didn't hear her. I only woke up a half-hour later, when Maura was banging things around in the kitchen and grumbling loudly enough to give the entire house a feeling of portentousness, as if windows might start breaking. Maura doesn't like getting up in the middle of the night—mostly because she has trouble getting back to sleep and so lies there more and more agitated by and fearful of not being rested enough in the morning—or, as she puts it, of not getting enough of an escape from herself. For her, sixteen straight hours of one's own self is enough. It's as if her mind is unionized, and there are very strict rules about when you're on duty and when you're not. Unfortunately, her poor body doesn't always cooperate. It's not uncommon for me to wake up at two o'clock and see the light on in the living room, where she is reading, helpless.

Being woken up at night now has to put the fear into her of what the near future holds.

Last night Maeve must've asked for warm milk with honey. That almost always puts her to sleep. (For Maura, it's a hefty glass of red wine, or cooking sherry if that's all we've got—but that's off-limits now.) I could tell by the slam of the refrigerator door that Maura wasn't happy with the request.

I pretended to be asleep when she came back to bed—not a generous decision but a self-protective one. I should've slung my arm over her and thanked her for getting up, but I was afraid that starting any conversation might delay both of us getting back to sleep.

And then, fifteen minutes later, Maeve padded in again. Maura pulled her onto her lap and hugged her tightly for a long time.

"Leave her here," I finally whispered. "You go sleep in her bed." That's what we did, and everyone—frustrated, embarrassed, exhausted—got another two hours.

Last night's fiasco reminded me of what has been, during the past five years, the single most disturbing part of parenthood for me: my tendency to use Maeve as a stand-in for Maura, to shower on her the attention it's been easier not to give to a complicated grown woman. Last night, rather than inch warily into the riled emotional state within Maura's head, it was so much easier to comfort Maeve, to ask her, after Maura had left the room, why she couldn't sleep (bad dream), and to snuggle with her while she dozed back off. The temptation to be satisfied with that misdirected attention has been so strong at times. It's gotten me into trouble, tension building up through days of growing resentments and holes dug deeper for me to sink into. So far, always, there has come the big release, the admonitions and realizations and accepted apologies.

One kid takes so much of our energy away from each other, makes it so much easier to think of each other merely as coworkers than as lovers. Our refrain is so often, "I never *see* you, except to give you Maeve or take her from you." And then we pledge to get babysitters, to have regular dates, to do more things all together. The resolution lasts for a while, and then of course dissipates, and we enter the cycle again.

It's impossible to guess how another kid thrown into the mix will help things. My very slim hope of an improvement lies in a passage I remember from an essay by Edward Hoagland, in which he observes that the poorer a family is, the more dogs it owns. One dog means being well-off. Four or five dogs means certain poverty. "Nobody got poor feeding a bunch of dogs, needless to say," Hoagland wrote, "because the more dogs a man had, the less he fed them." I've heard of similar things happening with children: parents of many children being more free because the kids, as Hoagland says of those dogs, forage as a pack and lead an existence of their own. Alas, I suspect it will take lots more than one additional kid to get us to that state of liberation.

JULY 26

The fact is, it's so much easier to be outwardly loving to a small child than it is to an adult. Maeve's always accepting of my affection, and there is no preparation period. In fact, she does at least half the work; she assumes, as only a five-year-old can, that all relationships are good and loving. She's lived by this even during those moments when she's tried out harsher sentiments, such as yesterday, when she wanted to watch a video and I said no, that she needed to go out in the backyard and play. "If you don't let me watch a video," she said, "I'll punch you in the stomach really hard." I held my arms up to give her a clear shot, and she took a swing, giggling the smallest bit under her seriousness. Then she got her game face back and told me, sternly, "Daddy, I don't like you anymore," and then her eyes got dreamy and she floated over and put her head against my hip and hugged my leg.

It'll get harder, of course. Adolescence lies ominously ahead.

JULY 29
Still on the lookout for that second-trimester magic. Maura's hormones seem less wild this time, or maybe it's just that whenever they do begin vibrating like electrons, Maeve will come running into the room, looking for someone to read a book to her.

JULY 30
Maeve's birthday party today. We had eight kids over, and they entertained themselves in the warm sunshine with the small blue plastic pool and the Slip 'n Slide. Maura tried without much success to get them enthused about a potato-sack race and the old egg-on-a-spoon race. She didn't even have much luck convincing them to dig banana slices out of plates of whipped cream with only their mouths, even though she and our friend Ann volunteered to go first. The kids looked on amused but completely unwilling to embarrass themselves in the same way. The hit of the party, I'll admit modestly, was the cake. I stayed up until three last night making it, a fact that Maeve loyally announced to each of her guests as they arrived. It's worthwhile having a kid who's impressed enough with my deeds to brag about them. And who's young enough to have friends who share her awe.

The cake was a Barbie doll in a big, wide dress. I'd driven across town to a store devoted completely to cake decorating, and I bought the mold — shaped like an inverted bowl — and a long-haired torso and head with a spike instead of legs. The saleslady, when I admitted that I'd never actually decorated a cake like this before (it became obvious when I didn't know the sizes of the pastry-bag tips), said, "Well, you sure picked a hard one to start with."

"As long as it has the vague shape of a doll," I said, knowing that the advantage to having a kid with imagination is that she'd fill in the gaps in my work, understand my *vision*.

I began baking after Maeve went to bed, and then at midnight, when the cake was cool enough, went at it with the pastry bags and a butter knife. The biggest challenge, artistically speaking, was the "bodice," which took on all kinds of interesting dimensions when I tried to spread the frosting over those little, plastic breasts. I ended up with something that looked feathery—stylish in a risqué prom dress kind of way.

It was hard to tell at the time because my eyes were so bleary, but the cake seemed to have turned out okay—the mauve ribbon around the bottom of the pink dress, the yellow flowers with their little white centers, the "beads" across the top of the bodice that actually looked more like a shark-tooth necklace. Still, when it was done the doll looked disconcertingly startled, because it oddly didn't have any top eyelashes and because its arms were sticking straight out. She was supposed to be holding a multicolored bouquet, but, you know, there's only so much a guy can do at 2:00 in the morning.

Anyway, Maeve saw it in the refrigerator in the morning and came running in to wake me and rave about how much she loved it. A tired but good start to the day.

The adults at the party joined the kids in oohing and ahhing with just the right tone and knowledgeable appreciation. I put off slicing into the cake for as long as I could. But once I did, and wedges of Barbie ended up on the pink paper plates, she tasted just as good as she had looked.

At the party, the parents sat in lawn chairs under the maple and ended up talking about getting the opposite of what you think you want in a kid. Our friend Kim said that when she found out she was having a girl, she was sure she didn't want to relive her own girlhood, but that she's had a blast doing it so far. And our friend Lynniece, whose son, Curtis, is one of Maeve's best buddies, desperately wanted a girl but has been shocked by how much fun it's been with a boy.

I'm ready to give up wishing for one thing or another. I'm almost even ready to whisper, or maybe just say silently to myself, I actually *want* a boy. Almost.

Why is it that I can get to that verge and then run into a story that pushes me backward one huge step? Mere hours after I wrote that line above, I was talking to an acquaintance about her boy, who is a few months older than Maeve and who sounds like one of my worst nightmares. Do I go in search of this bad propaganda in order to keep myself safe? To bolster my old beliefs, solidify my prejudices? I don't know, but the images this woman shared were almost too disturbing for words, and I've been trying since to understand what she *really* meant when she said that her son is not at all mean, but that if he saw something he wanted, he wouldn't hesitate to grab it out of some other kid's hands and shove that kid to the ground. Is this the "boys will be boys" rationale?

On the other hand, the woman said that her mother tells her she was exactly the same when she was a kid—and so obviously there's something besides gender at work there. This woman said she now apologizes to her mother every single time she sees her. It sounds like parenthood for her has become a mixture of shock and shame. And yet she seems to like the kid. Go figure.

JULY 31

A robin has built a nest in the hanging petunia on the front porch and has been sitting there the last couple of days warming a single blue egg. There's not much privacy in that location, and when the wind blows the pot swings back and forth and twists from side to side, but she doesn't seem to mind, not even when Lila, our younger cat, sprawls on the porch and looks out the tops of her eyes at her. We've been checking every hour or so to make sure Mommy-Bird is still there, and it's added a small bit of drama to the doldrums of Maura's own pregnancy. We can see the bird's head and tail feathers above the flowers and leaves, and she's sitting there with a stately zen-ness. I like to think she was drawn to that site by the pregnancy vibes flowing out of the house.

After watching her for two days, I wondered aloud to Maura whether the bird might be bored, or whether she was in some state of bliss.

"That's what parenthood is, isn't it?" she said. "An oscillation between boredom and blissfulness?"

I talked to my friend Karl last night, whose little boy, John, is way off the scale of cuteness. Several of us have already planned his and Maeve's wedding. Karl reported that John has taken a sudden and intense interest in things that shoot — guns, bows and arrows, slingshots, straws and spitwads. I've read enough about these transformations to accept readily that it's inevitable, maybe even healthy in an anachronistically evolutionary way. But we're going to be visiting them this weekend, and we'll just have to see whether John is still marrying material, or whether he's shot himself right out of the running.

Talking with Karl reminded me of an Art Spiegelman comic in which a father wants to get his little daughter to play with something besides dolls — the endless nurturing is driving him nuts — and so he buys her a fire truck and shows her how it can zoom around the room and make all kinds of loud noises. The strip ends with her cradling the fire truck in her lap and rocking it to sleep.

Maeve has finally learned how she scares Maura when she comes into our room in the middle of the night and puts her fingers on Maura's face. So now she announces herself: "It's your daughter."

In the dark, emerging blearily from a deep sleep, the pronouncement is like something from a strange movie.

AUGUST 1

How does one prepare to fall in love again? And how, especially, when the creature I'm expecting to fall in love with doesn't even exist yet? The oddness of that experience with Maeve is still fresh to me — the knowledge that I would love whatever came along, without having a helpful clue of what, beyond the obvious, it would be. And that I immediately did love her so much. This time, I'm wondering how to stay fresh for it, how not to go through it with a seasoned knowingness.

AUGUST 2

So far this weekend, the little boy John seems like a good, sensible kid. It's early Saturday morning right now, and I can hear him and Maeve downstairs talking about which board games they have. John is expounding on the virtues of Chutes and Ladders. The civilized segment of his brain seems in control this morning. The gun part will probably wake up around noon, like a teenager.

We took a drive through the country later in the morning, and then stopped for lunch at a diner in a small, blue-collar town. Coincidentally, to go along with our running conversation about guns so far this weekend, there was taped to the wall above our table a flyer inviting kids eight to thirteen years old to a "meat shoot." Such an event must be just as ritualistic and normal as a birthday party at Chuck E. Cheese is in the suburbs. Maybe—I dare say—healthier.

John's dad, Karl, is adamant about not giving John any toy guns, but he *is* thinking about buying him a real gun—a .22—sometime soon in order to "teach him how guns work." I'm not sure I see the logic there, but then I'm a citified liberal who's never actually shot anything more powerful than a pellet gun. Karl claims to have gone hunting when he was a kid.

Also, he's a psychologist, and so thinks out the subconscious causes and ramifications of these kinds of dilemmas. Here's his lesson for this weekend: A boy is afraid of losing something—the castration fear—and so becomes aggressive in order to head off that loss. Hence, teach him how to shoot in a real but controlled environment, and thereby help to tame his aggression, or at least funnel it into nonviolent outlets. I was abstractly empathizing with his trouble, but really thankful I didn't have to deal with it myself, when he turned the tables on me, arguing that if we *don't* teach Maeve how to use a gun, we may be missing an opportunity to show her how to use and be comfortable with aggression. It could be a boxing-in that's limiting in its own way.

Now, this is an issue that has occurred to Maura and me: How to encourage Maeve to be more healthfully aggressive—not on the firing range or in the woods during squirrel season, but, say, in groups of other kids. She's no pushover, but there are moments when she'll step back from a confrontation or refuse to say aloud what she really thinks. I prefer to think of this as an early wisdom, because who really needs to get into the face of any five-year-old who acts his age? Maura points out, however, that this is Maeve's world, and these are the people she's going to have to be jockeying with all her life. Might as well begin now to perfect a wide range of tools for dealing with them.

The thing is, Maeve's never asked for a gun, has never pretended that a stick is a gun, and probably wouldn't agree to shoot a gun if I handed it to her. I suspect that getting her at all interested in a gun would be as difficult as getting John *un*interested. This'll probably be what they'll fight about most once they're married.

AUGUST 3

Maura had the football dream last night. She was supposed to play for the local college team, and she kept insisting to them that she couldn't, that she was pregnant.

I think she woke up with the same feeling of helpless desperation I did after I had my own football dream.

In this morning's paper was a quote from a baseball player on the Seattle Mariners. It seems that wives of the players have given birth to seven sons so far this summer, and the latest player to be so blessed said, crassly, "I'll take it. That's one less wedding I have to pay for." Maybe he said it just because he had to say something. Maybe it was humor among the guys. Even so, comments like that make *me* want to have a daughter, as a counterbalance to such imbecility.

This afternoon Maeve said, "Mommy, I really want a girl baby. I'm going to pray for one tonight."

And I thought, well, a five-year-old girl's prayers probably carry some weight.

Maeve is the only locus of certainty in this house now.

AUGUST 4

All the way to Pennsylvania and back this weekend, Maura and I floated possible names around the car, without much luck. We must've gone through eight or ten dozen of them, and would've gone through more if we'd remembered to bring the baby-name books with us. During some stretches we were reduced to free-associating from road signs and billboards ("How about Merge? Marge?" "How about Dewdrop?"), and we tried to reconstruct our family trees, to remember—if we ever knew—the middle names of great uncles and aunts. Maeve weighed in on whichever ones struck her as especially good or inane, and when she added her own suggestions, like Bullwinkle, we reminded her that when it comes right down to it, she's likely to be outvoted, 2 to 1.

By the time we were rolling back into Syracuse, we had two or three girls' names we each felt some tepid attraction to, and absolutely no overlap on the boys' side.

Tonight at dinner Maeve said, in her white-lab-coat voice, "I hope this one doesn't cramp up and die like the other ones." I had to get the applesauce from the refrigerator anyway, and so let Maura handle the response. I think there was a soothing reassurance, then a transition I missed, and then, as I sat back down, Maura was saying, "You can't have a baby without a daddy." (Had I denied responsibility?)

Uh oh, I thought.

"You can't have a baby without a daddy?" Maeve asked.

"What you need," Maura said, "is an egg and a sperm," and then she put down her own fork and began an enthusiastic explanation, with lots of emphasis — it seemed to me — on how special it was that the egg only comes down the tube once a month, while billions of sperm loiter around constantly. She verbally diagrammed some of the physiology, the internal structures, and then began quizzing Maeve.

"Who has the egg?" Maura said excitedly.

"You do!" Maeve shouted.

"And who has the sperm?"

"Daddy does!"

They went on this way for a good minute or two. Then Maeve began considering the mechanics. "How does the sperm get in there?" she asked.

"It swims," Maura said.

"No, I mean, how does it get in your belly?"

"Well, Daddy puts his penis in my vagina."

"Huh?!" Maeve shouted, her face opened in surprise like a koala bear's.

"It's something married people do," Maura said, suddenly deciding that she'd reached a sufficient level of specificity.

"But how?" Maeve asked. She'd recovered and wanted details.

"As you get older, dear, things will become more clear about this," Maura said. It was a brush-off that didn't have much chance of working. It didn't.

"I want to watch," Maeve said.

"No no no no no," Maura said. "No no no no no."

Maeve laughed. "Just kidding."

She went over to the digesting chair—an overstuffed chair we keep in the kitchen and which she named months ago, after we instituted a new rule that we all had to sit and digest and talk for fifteen minutes after eating—and began singing to herself. I whispered to Maura, "Hey, I thought we had a few more years, but now *that's* done."

AUGUST 5

When I mentioned the sperm-egg conversation to a friend later—a guy who has a daughter—we slipped into the topic of future boyfriends and the fact that they'll be bringing penises along with them and wanting to follow the mechanics that Maura had described to Maeve. My friend's face scrunched up and he said, "And I'll beat the shit out of them."

I used to *thrive* on jealousy, and it doesn't take much effort to rake up that old feeling, in the way I can remember the pain from a kidney stone or the frustration of being shy. It strikes me as strange, therefore, that, at the moment, at least, I *don't* want to beat the shit out of Maeve's future lovers, that I find it hard to relate to the line I used to accept as part of the drill of being a father—that I wouldn't let any daughter of mine date until she'd, say, finished grad school. I don't think I've related to that line since I actually *had* a daughter. Now, the idea of Maeve, way off in the future, being sexual actually gives me comfort, like the idea of her being intellectual. I have no idea why this is, unless it's because she's such a physical person now, so quick to hug and snuggle, to wrap her arms around Maura and say, "I want to smell your neck." When I fall asleep with her, she slings her leg over my hip in a carefree sprawl.

My friend Stephanie once pointed out how insane it is that we give kids all kinds of physical affection until they're two or three, and then we make them sleep completely by themselves for the next fifteen or twenty years, after which they have to make the transition back on their own. I don't know what the solution to that is. God knows that family beds have had their ugly histories. But what I want is for Maeve to remain physical in some healthy and safe way all through her childhood and teenage years, for her to grow slowly and confidently into a mature sex life. I even told Maura once that I hope we can talk with Maeve, some day, about how important it is to be passionate as a lover, but Maura looked at me as if I were more naïve than she'd ever realized, and said that *no* girl would want to hear that stuff from her parents. We'll see when that conversation comes up. The way things are going, it may be next week.

Maeve's been going to a town-sponsored playground in the mornings for the last couple of weeks, and this morning they had a "talent show," which I put in quotations because I have some doubts about lip-synching to a rap song being talent. What put a knot in my stomach, though, was the modeling—the older girls sashaying out and striking poses. Maura leaned over to me and whispered, "Whose idea was *this?*"

I kept telling myself: *It's only a playground, run by a bunch of college kids, don't be so PC.* I kept looking to see how Maeve was reacting. (Her group had done "Old McDonald," lame enough in its own five-minutes-of-rehearsal kind of way, but comfortably innocent.) I was happy that she had a confused look on her face, rather than anything approaching fascination.

It got me thinking that I don't really know anything about girls yet, that the real education is yet to come, and that all I know so far is what it's like to raise one very well-behaved and very young child who just happens to be a girl and whose major interests lean toward girlish things. At the moment, I feel just the tiniest bit of trepidation.

AUGUST 6

The middle trimester is low-key. Maura can often feel the baby kicking, but I've never been able to rush to her belly before it stops. So I just watch her getting bigger. She's begun walking around with her hands cupped under her belly, like an old man, or someone carrying a load of firewood.

Now would be about the time we'd be having the amnio and tri-beta tests if we'd gone that route. But the opportunities for them are passing, and I feel a little melancholy as they go by. I think it's only because they would add some excitement to the days, like we get when Maura has a check-up.

AUGUST 7

I've been feeling grumpy all week, possessive of my time alone—of which, it seems to me, I've had none. This house is small, and every time I go into a room by myself, Maura or Maeve walks through. Worse, I've been looking at Maura's belly and thinking there are many other things I could be doing in the next five years besides raising a baby. I could write, for one, or take more trips to New York City, or . . . have some time alone. I've been jealous of my childless friends, and the ones whose kids are grown and out of the house. When you have kids in your forties, lots of your friends have kids who are out of the house. I read once about a favorite writer of mine who is so protective of her writing study that her husband hasn't even entered it. Needless to say, she doesn't have kids.

We've got an old shed in the backyard that I've been planning to turn into a writing studio. It's next summer's project—if I'm not with the kid all the time. Since we bought this old house, I've inched my way through several big projects, doing a couple of hours here or there, rarely getting the chance to work a full day straight. Projects tend to take months rather than days. When the projects haven't involved power saws, I've tried to get Maeve in the swing of things, letting her go at it with a paint roller. It's not time-efficient, but at least we're on task. Lately, rather than daydreaming about how I'm going to line my new writing studio with maple bookshelves and cut a big picture window in the south wall, I've been thinking about the best way to keep the door locked.

I was in this mood yesterday when I found out that a friend of mine—a guy my age who has one small kid and who, with his wife, has gone through the same agonizing decision-making in the last couple of years that Maura and I did about whether to draw again from the deck or hold with the hand they've got—had a vasectomy this week. The news put a knot in my stomach. First there was the visceral reaction. I always feel faint at the thought of the procedure, and I have to gorge on candy and donuts to get my blood sugar back up. Beyond that, though, I was also thinking about this other path we could've taken, and I felt a little Robert Frost-ish with uncertainty. Fortunately, that only lasted a minute, after which I actually felt good about Maura's pregnancy again—better than I'd felt all week—as if now that I knew someone going down that other road, I could plod along on the one we'd chosen.

When I visited my friend at his house, it was clear—even if he was a little slow in bending down to pick out a video for his daughter—that *he* was happy about his own decision. No surprise there. Months ago, he and his wife had given us literature on the intelligence and social adaptability of only-children. We'd read the articles, but they'd actually gone out and dug them up. Once you get to that stage, you're probably just looking for evidence to support a decision you've already made. More power to them. Their daughter will be starting kindergarten next year, and they'll have *all kinds of time alone.*

AUGUST 8

Here's some news. My youngest brother, Steve, who just turned forty and has three daughters under five, the youngest not even crawling yet, is going to be a grandfather. Two months ago he had his own vasectomy to stop the madness of his own procreation, but he now flies right into some different kind of parental experience. I sense he has mixed feelings about it.

The new father-to-be is Steve's twenty-year-old son, Ryan, who was born when Steve was nineteen. We've all watched Ryan grow up to be one of the nicest people you can imagine—sweet, sensitive, entirely giving. His younger cousins like to hang on him, and I think they constitute a fairly vibrant fan club. Ryan's one of those kids whose high school portrait you put on your refrigerator and babysitters come into the kitchen and want to know who *that* is.

It's almost impossible to imagine how different it will be for Ryan and his girlfriend Karen to be raising a newborn than it is now for Steve and Jeanne and will be soon for Maura and me. Biologically, I suppose, twenty or twenty-one is when you should be having a baby, because the hormones are pumping and the muscles are limber. You've got your wind. Beyond that, as Steve well knows, the advantages are slim.

AUGUST 9

So, I was lying in bed this morning at 6:00 and some punk parked his car in the street a few houses down with the radio playing really loudly. He opened the door and left it open while he went to someone's house. He was gone several minutes, long enough for a full song. I got up and peered angrily out the window. And I thought that when Maeve is eighteen years old and pulling pranks like that, I'll be almost sixty, probably completely unable to stomp out there and give her no-good friends a lesson in manners. The guy finally drove off and I slumped back into bed. But I was disgusted enough that I couldn't go back to sleep, and so I got up and ran four miles, just to send a message to all the guys who are going to be hovering noisily around our house in twelve or thirteen years.

Maura revealed last night that she has the feeling the baby is going to be a girl. No concrete reason why—just a feeling. She was rubbing her belly absently, the way she rubs the cat.

"And how does that make you feel?" I asked.

"Good," she said, smiling.

"Good," I said, remembering that for a long time she was sure that Maeve was going to be a boy, because she was carrying low.

AUGUST 10

Choosing a name is a fragile process. Whenever one occurs to me that I might like, I have to let it roll around in my head for a while, waiting for it to sort of come together like a ball of bread dough, before I mention it even to Maura. It's only then that it might withstand some outside poking and punching down, though many times it doesn't. Most of the time I say it aloud and hear the polite silence from Maura, see the nod of the head, and I realize how misguided I've been, as if I've almost painted the living room purple. But she hits on just as many that make me wonder where her mind's at, and so we just plow on, leaving unusable names behind us like litter.

Every few weeks the local paper prints the names of babies born recently in the county. I read the latest list aloud to Maura this morning. It's good to find out what to avoid because of overpopularity or because—like Destiny Angel Star—they're the product of a couple of eighteen-year-old minds. One boy was named Thunder, which I thought was ballsy. There were a number of names for which we both nodded and said, "That's not too bad." But picking a name from the vital statistics feels a little like running out to get the same shirt your neighbor just bought. Not that I didn't add a few of these to our list. And not that I don't frequently read the phone book looking for more.

I had a dream last night that a friend of ours — it wasn't someone we actually know in real life — had a four-month-old boy whom she hadn't named yet. She was getting pressure from all sides, but she didn't care in the least. She'd give him a name when she'd decided on one. I woke up really liking her.

On a walk today, I told Maeve that we should stop in and visit my friend Les. Maeve had once met him briefly, but my descriptions of what he looked like weren't helping her place him. So she got right to the heart of how we identify many adults to her. "Is he somebody's father or something?" she asked.

"No, he doesn't have any kids."

"Why not?"

"I don't know. I guess he decided not to have any."

"But," she said, "who does he put to bed?"

The mind of the five-year-old is amazingly supple and creative, at the same time that it's driven by the realities of its own experience.

AUGUST 11

I asked Maeve what aspect of the new baby excites her most. She thought for a minute, then said, "I'll have a new friend."

Yesterday she and I were hanging out, taking that walk, then resting on the bed and reading some books and singing some songs, later joking around about cow poop in the backyard while I was putting manure around the tomato and pepper plants, and the word that kept floating through my mind was *friend friend friend*. It was one of the most comforting sensations of parenthood that I can remember.

Maura was lying in bed last night with her hands on her belly and exclaiming as if the baby was doing a karate demonstration in there. Then it would stop, and she'd say, "She's eight or ten inches long now, so she can't hide forever." Then the kid would move and Maura would jump again as if she'd been goosed.

So I lay my hand across her belly, letting Maura move it to the most likely spot. It was a long minute and a half before something bulged up into my palm.

"*There's* its little butt," I said.

Maura glowed. "Or its head," she said.

It was nice to finally get physical evidence, but the experience was also like whale-watching, in that once you see what you came for, you're ready to head back to shore.

Maura said that Maeve asked her this morning, while they were sitting in the kitchen, "So, has Daddy already put his penis up your vagina?"

Maura was a little taken aback, both by the preposition—she hadn't originally described it as *up* but as *in*—and by the fact that it had been several days since the facts of life had been mentioned.

"Uh, yes," Maura admitted.

"When?" Maeve wanted to know.

"Well, back in April, I think?"

Maeve nodded. "But I didn't watch because I'm not supposed to."

"Right," Maura agreed.

"When did he do it for me?" she asked.

"I think that was November, dear. But, you know, almost six years ago."

Ah, the pieces are falling into place, the timelines and acts of responsibility emerging.

AUGUST 12

Maura has taken to calling the baby "she." I warned her that this is a brash and dangerous assumption, but she does it anyway. When she was cooing to it that way in bed last night, I suddenly had a flashback to the first few Christmases I spent at Maura's mom's house in Vermont. I would be there with Maura, her sisters Jennifer and Sheila, her mom, her Aunt Brigid, and her Great Aunt Olive. Me and half a dozen females. We used to sit around the fireplace, and everyone would be knitting except me. Most of the time it was comforting, but every few hours the gentle domesticity of the place—the clicking of knitting needles, the almost absentminded soft laughter, the stillness—got to me so badly that I had to take the dog (the only other male around) for a long walk through the snow. Every couple of days the dog and I would climb a 1250-foot mountain that overlooks the town, and from the summit we'd be able to see the house and the smoke coming from the chimney. I could feel the domesticity from up there, and I'd tell the dog we had to take the long way home. We'd be out so long that he'd get those little ice balls in the fur of his paws and have to limp until we'd take a break and I'd melt them with my cold hands. Other times, I simply went into the other room and watched football on TV.

It occurs to me now and then that if we have another daughter, we will have to get a dog.

Last night we were talking about children's songs, and Maura reminded Maeve of one that always used to make Maeve cry. It's the one about the barnyard that goes, "Oh, I had a pig and the pig had me," and you go through all the animals and make the noises as obnoxiously as you can then end each verse with "fiddle-eye-fee." Maura began to sing it right there.

"I hated that song too," I said. "And you just kept singing it."

"It amused me," Maura said. "I thought we'd all grow to love it."

"But we only grew to hate it more," I said.

AUGUST 13

Well, George W. Bush has sent out his $400 tax-refund checks for people with kids — or at least some people with kids — and when we got ours, Maura insisted we send the money immediately to Howard Dean. I'm all for it, though the check is still sitting on the kitchen counter, calling out: *Buy new tires with me!*

Then the family issue of the *New Yorker* arrived in the mail today, and I was certainly happy to read that "having a child is now the best indicator of whether someone will end up in financial collapse." The sentences following that were just as uplifting: "Married couples with children are twice as likely as childless couples to file for bankruptcy. They're seventy-five percent more likely to be late paying their bills. And they're also far more likely to face foreclosure on their homes. Most of these people are not, by the usual standards, poor. They're middle-class couples who are in deep financial trouble in large part because they have kids."

We're so middle-class we've got a white picket fence (in need of paint). Of course we long ago left the ranks of the childless, and so I guess we fall in between the people furthest away from bankruptcy and the people with "kids." But we'll soon step into that vortex.

Every once in a while, during our deliberations about having another kid, Maura or I would ask, "Can we *afford* this?" And the answer was pretty much always the same: no idea. At the moment, yeah, we could scrape up enough money to buy diapers and maybe a few of those plastic things infants chew on when they're teething. During the first year, especially if you're breast-feeding—which Maura did with Maeve and plans to do again—that's about the extent of the day-to-day expenses. Then if this kid turns out to be a girl, she'll wear all of Maeve's old clothes and we'll catch a break there. They can share a room, and we won't have to build an addition. (We're short on rooms.) If it's a boy, well, he doesn't get as many clothes and he sleeps in a tent in the backyard. It was pretty easy to imagine that we could get the new kid to five years old just as adequately as we've gotten Maeve there, barring any disastrous medical expenses. When I tried to imagine the years after that, it was like taking my glasses off.

Anyway, as the *New Yorker* pointed out, it's not diapers that will eat up your paychecks. It's housing and education. The housing's steep because houses are bigger these days and because everyone—surprise—wants to live in a safe neighborhood with good public schools. And the education is steep because college tuition goes up. We've got an education fund for Maeve, though it doesn't grow much because she's really lousy about sending any money into it. I suppose she would expect us to do that, if she even knew the fund existed. But it's kind of down at the bottom of the possible places to put whatever spare money there is, and so it maybe gets a small infusion once a year, just to make us feel we're being responsible planners. What we're really doing is counting on her smarts to get her a full ride someplace. That's responsible, right?

With the numbers you read about the future of college tuition anyway—what'll it be? a million a year or something by the time Maeve goes, plus textbooks and beer?—I just don't see how we could save enough anyhow. It's too daunting. Maura's been out of college for a long time, and she's still paying $200 a month in student loans, and will be for a several more years.

In her room Maeve's got this three-foot-high plastic ice cream cone that's actually a bank. I usually throw my spare change in there, and right now the thing's half full. I doubt it contains more than a hundred bucks, since lots of it is pennies. But for a long time we had a rule that we could never take any coins *out* of the cone. When it got full, we'd deposit the money in the real bank and send a check for that amount to the real college fund. Then we had a couple of emergencies in which we needed just a dollar or three—a field trip at preschool, for instance, that we didn't remember until the morning of. So we dipped. And then Maeve began dipping, not to spend the money but to carry some around in her Hello Kitty purse and use it as another toy. The sanctified seal on the bank got broken. Now I'm not sure there's much holiness to the cone at all. The other night when we decided to walk to the corner and get some real ice cream cones at the Sno-Top, we dug out five bucks in quarters. When you start pilfering the quarters rather than the nickels and dimes, your whole balance goes to hell fast.

The robin drama has had a bad ending. Last Sunday when I checked the nest, there were three newly hatched babies in there. When I checked again on Monday, there was only one. I looked all over the ground under the nest, but the babies were nowhere, and the only conclusion I could reach was that big, bad nature got them. Then the momma bird stopped coming by a couple days ago, and the nest has sat empty. What happened to the last baby is anyone's guess, though it didn't look anywhere near old enough to get out on its own. There's a general feeling of sadness around here for momma bird. I took down the dead plant and removed the nest and set that on the wicker table on the porch as a memorial.

AUGUST 16

Maeve and I took my sister, my brother-in-law, and their two daughters to New York City this week, and one of the highlights for the girls was spending a couple of hours on the rides at Wolfman Rink in Central Park. It was evening and not crowded, so the girls could jump on any ride they wanted and stay on for as long as they wanted. Still, a couple of times when Maeve was in line one boy or another would cut in front of her, and I actually found myself grabbing the shoulders of their shirts to hold them back while Maeve went ahead. I missed one kid and he plowed ahead of us onto the roller coaster. He sat a few cars in front of us and every time we'd go around a curve he'd twist his head back and stare at us like some wax-museum mummy. I thought, *You little crew-cut snot.*

One of the lowlights of the trip was when the electricity went out, not only in the city but all over the northeast. We were on the Staten Island Ferry at the time, and when we got back to Manhattan, subways weren't running, busses were overflowing, and there wasn't a taxi to be had. Even if there was, traffic was going nowhere fast. The only way we could get back to our car on 59th Street was to walk. It took us three hours, and most of the time it felt like we were swimming against the current, and I carried Maeve all but a total of two blocks. Maeve has many, many talents, but at this stage of the game, walking very far is not one of them. I've tried hard not to scare her with threats about how life might change for her once the new baby comes, but along about 45th Street, when I'd switched her for the fiftieth time from my shoulders to my right arm to piggyback, I said, a bit harshly, "You know, when the baby comes you're not going to get carried anymore, because I'm going to be carrying the baby instead." This seemed to surprise her, but she thought for a minute and said, "Mommy can carry the baby, and you can still carry me."

It reminded me of her logic from last winter, when we were trying to get her to wipe herself after peeing, a task we knew she could do perfectly well because she did it at preschool. "But," she said when we argued that there should be no difference between school and home, "you're my parents. It's your *job* to take care of me."

AUGUST 17

My right ankle and right hip hurt, and it must be from having carried Maeve halfway across Manhattan the other day. I'm tempted to tell Maura that I can currently empathize with her own carrying of a child, but there's really not often a good time to make such a comment.

The dog is back in the house. This is Calvin, Maura's mom's collie. Gail went on a cruise across the Atlantic, and so we get the dog and Gail's car for two weeks. ("Enjoy being a two-car family," Gail told me when I dropped her off at the airport, and the extra wheels will be convenient.) Calvin is not any healthier than the last time we took care of him — still ancient and stiff, and again Gail said that she'd understand if we had to take any drastic action while she was gone.

We'll do our best, try to be more successful sitters than the one our friend Renee hired recently. Renee asked a friend to feed her budgie while she was away, but the friend forgot for a week, and when she finally remembered she rushed over to Renee's apartment and found the bird dead at the bottom of its cage. The friend felt horrible enough that she didn't even make up a story about the bird having a heart attack or anything.

AUGUST 18

Had a nineteen-week checkup with the OB today, and the heartbeat was as easy to find as the pulse on someone who's just sprinted the 440. The checkup was brief and the doc again pronounced Maura "perfect in every way."

I wondered aloud when we might have an ultrasound.

"Curious about what's in there?" he said, smiling.

I shrugged.

"Don't you routinely do an ultrasound at twenty-eight weeks?" Maura asked.

"Nothing is ever 'routine,'" the doctor corrected her, in the same way a furniture salesman once told us that we didn't want to find chairs that *matched* a used cherry dining-room table we'd bought but ones that *blended*. The doctor smiled with the pleasure of a man who knows the loopholes in a touchy and bureaucratic health industry. "If it's 'routine,' insurance doesn't pay for it. Instead, we have" — he dropped his voice as if he were dictating what to write on the insurance form — "'a woman of advanced maternal age with a previous abnormal pregnancy and we need to find out how the fetus is developing.' We'll make an appointment for two weeks out."

"Finally, an advantage to being old," Maura said.

"You're perfect," the doctor said.

AUGUST 19

Last night Maeve wanted to read *Making Life* before bed — the latest book on pregnancy we've gotten from the library. On one page Maeve pointed to a picture of a sperm worming its way into the egg and said, "And there's the sperm the egg has chosen. Mommy told me that."

"I'm sure she did," I said, recalling an article Maura likes to have the students in her Literature and Science class read about who's really in charge at the moment of conception. I wondered what Maura would say to a son.

AUGUST 20

For the last few days I've felt depressed and grumpy. I think I've said a total of five words to Maura. I haven't asked about the Very Young Elvis or put my hand on Maura's belly. I see her walking through the kitchen and think, Why are you pregnant? My lower back hurts, I've had a headache for two days, and I only want to go on a long drive by myself—to, say, Manitoba.

My friend Mike called this morning and asked if I wanted to play tennis, and if I didn't care about embarrassing myself I would've said, "Yeah, in ten years, when the kids can stay by themselves for five goddamn minutes." Maura sensed my frustration and promised to try to find a babysitter for a few hours this afternoon, but she later confessed that she'd struck out.

I don't know where the tension is coming from. It's probably that Maura and I both start teaching next week and have a lot of prep to do, I haven't exercised in three weeks, and I'm feeling as if I've done nothing but take care of people for the past two weeks—starting with having to get all the family out of Manhattan during the blackout. This is stupid, because at the time it was actually weirdly *fun*. So was the company. It's only when it's all over that the resentment bubbles like hot tar. I was so bitter last night at dinner that I didn't even say anything when Maura poured herself a small glass of wine. I thought, *Go ahead and brain-damage the baby! Who cares?*

AUGUST 21

Well, shit. There's nothing that puts a bad mood more into perspective than having your cat die. That's what happened yesterday. It was Perry, the cat we've had for ten years. Maura came downstairs in the late afternoon to find him stretched out in the mudroom on his side, not long dead but definitely gone. Just an hour or two before, he'd been as healthy as ever. It must've been his heart, his lungs, something that would fail and kill him quickly.

Maeve and I got home a little while later. Maura could barely whisper to me, "Perry's dead"—words to which, on a sunny and relatively carefree afternoon, there seems no imaginable immediate response. None of us really knew what we ought to do. Maura had already put Perry on the wicker chair on the front porch, and so we went out there to see him. He looked to me as if he were sleeping there as he always has, but Maeve was more observant and honest and said that he didn't look at all like he was sleeping. He looked dead. She said it was because his lips had sunk in around his teeth. She was right. We petted him for a while, and then I carried him to the back patio and lay him on the table there. Maura brought Lila, the other cat, over, to let her smell Perry and know for herself what had happened, but she wasn't having any of it. She zipped off and we didn't see her for hours. If she understood, she wasn't going to stand around and be sentimental about it.

We buried him in a good spot in the backyard, behind the perennial bed, where there's some privacy but also some sun and space to plant a memorial tree next spring.

Maeve takes these things so well, it seems. She didn't cry, but once or twice when I was digging the grave she said, "I'm going inside, this is making me too sad." It could also have been the mosquitoes. But she stroked Perry as he lay on the fluffy oval pet bed that we'd bury him on, and she told him what a wonderful cat he'd been. It was her idea to put a can of wet food in the grave with him, and it was Maura's idea to put in his leash, his brush, and his ear mite drops. ("It's how I cared for him," she explained, "and he might need them on the other side.") Maeve helped shovel the dirt back into the hole. Later, she said, "You know one good thing about Perry being dead? Now we won't have to keep him from going outside."

"Yes, he'll always be outside," I said.

We spent much of the evening reminiscing and having a beer in Perry's honor. (Maura sipped.) Maura cried a lot, and I wanted to but didn't. My chest was heavy. We had dinner only because Maeve needed to eat.

"Do you think he and Patricia are together now?" Maura asked, thinking of our friend who died last month of leukemia. Patricia had lived around the corner from us when we'd gotten Perry. Maura and I didn't know much about cats at the time, and we'd given Perry his first flea bath by holding him in the empty tub and pouring water over him. It was slippery and awkward and painful for all—sort of like a bad game of Twister—but we survived it with a small sense of bungled accomplishment. To make up for the bath, I suggested we treat him to a blow-drying, which I'd recently read many cats love. "I'll hold him and you dry him," I told Maura, but when she turned on her dryer—a small and high-pitched one—it scared Perry so badly that his back claws dug long lines down the insides of my forearms and he twisted his head around and sunk his teeth through the end of my index finger. I watched them go right through my skin. I dropped him, we banged around trying to open the bathroom door, and Maura was screaming. Five seconds later, Perry sat heaving on the carpet in the hallway, I was holding my bleeding arms over the sink, and Maura looked as if she might faint. We were all embarrassed.

A couple of weeks later, Patricia, who had once worked in a vet's office, offered to bathe Perry, and she did it in the kitchen sink, holding his front paws between her fingers and doing everything with calm confidence. Perry melted in her hands, even resting his head on her forearm as she soaped him up. It was an amazing sight, and it taught us how to treat this cat.

"Patricia's probably giving him a bath right now," I said.

One of the hardest parts of Perry's death is that he won't be here to see the new baby. He was so good last time, jumping up on Maeve's changing table to lick her head and get her to stop crying.

"With mixed results," Maura pointed out, smiling.

"It's hard to imagine having a baby *at all* without Perry around," I said. I had been imagining bringing a baby into the very circumstances we've created around us—repeating, in fact, the very circumstances we'd created for Maeve. Can there really be a member of our family who will not have known Perry? We got him a month after our honeymoon, and from then on he was there every moment of our marriage, every moment of Maeve's life.

"He would've liked it," Maura whispered. "He would've found it all very interesting."

She gave a slight laugh and recalled the time she'd had her wisdom teeth out and Perry climbed into bed with her and put his head on the pillow next to her. "I'm afraid sometimes he was better at empathy than we are," she said.

"He had it over me in spades," I said.

This was not simply our own opinion. Perry collected similar compliments throughout his life, and maybe we'll make a little headstone for him with our favorite. It came from Mrs. Pearson of South Dakota, who stayed in our house in Iowa City once when we were out of town and she was visiting her son. She wasn't a cat person, but Perry charmed her, and she left us a note that said, "Perry is a sweet and polite cat." Indeed he was.

"If I had known he was going to die in August, I would've let him outside," Maura said, her lip quivering.

"There was no way to know."

We sat and talked, not only about Perry but about how unpleasant the last few days have been, mostly thanks to my mood. Maura told me how crazy it makes her not to feel close to me, and I apologized for taking a mental break in a way that put her in a bad mood, too. And for the fact that it took the death of our cat to ease the tension.

That cat added a lot of mellowness to our lives, right to the end.

AUGUST 22

More crying today. It was Maeve this time, and it was because she had to get three shots before starting kindergarten. She was so excited about visiting the doctor before that — telling the doctor who her teacher will be, laughing when the doctor tapped on her knee and her leg sprung forward, exclaiming "Oh boy!" and giggling when the doctor put the cold stethoscope on her back. When all the fun stuff was done, though, and she found out she had to have shots, she curled up in Maura's lap and begged, in the most pitiful voice, "Don't let them give me shots." It was heartbreaking, though not as heartbreaking as when I had to hold her down so she could get the first shot in her thigh and then hold her in my arms so she could get another shot in each of her arms. She screamed, flailed. A second nurse had to come in and assist.

When the evil nurses left, Maeve huddled next to Maura and found the strength to talk to the baby about the shots. Beforehand, we had tried to calm her down by saying that she needed to teach the baby how to handle shots — a manipulation transparent even to a five-year-old.

Still, she humored us. Half crying, she spoke into Maura's belly: "Baby, when you get shots it's going to hurt, but only for a little while. Can you be brave, Baby? You can get Barbie Band-Aids like I have."

Then later this evening, Maeve told me, in a voice of calm impartiality, "You know, even though the shots hurt some, I kind of liked them. They were interesting." She began giving them to her stuffed animals, exhorting them into fearlessness.

AUGUST 23

I can hardly go in the backyard without getting a lump in my throat and feeling so sad about Perry. The grass is long, but I'm letting it grow, so as not to disturb him for a few days. Each evening I go out there to say good night and lay a fresh sprig of catnip on his grave. It's mawkish, I know, but I do it anyway.

Maura, who used to be a waitress and at times of stress has dreams that she has to work that kind of job again, had a dream last night that she was waiting tables, and standing over by the front door watching her was Perry.

"Did he want a table?" I asked.

"No," she said, "but it made me feel better just to know he was there."

Well, Maeve's changed her tune. She's begun telling people that she wants a brother rather than a sister. "Why?" I asked, completely surprised.

"With a brother, I won't have to share all my dresses," she explained. "I want to keep them until I grow out of them."

And yet the other day in the children's section at the library, I overheard her having a conversation with another five-year-old girl in which she said, very clearly, "I like girls better than boys."

It's a good thing for all of us that we don't have any choice in this matter. And that in two weeks we'll find out.

AUGUST 24

Even by this point, the lurking dangers of the first couple months of pregnancy feel far away. The chance of a miscarriage at this stage is probably near zero, and the Marfan's fiasco is just an annoying memory, though I still hold it against that doctor for being so alarmist. It's sort of my SOP to approach all things in the calmest manner possible, so much so that I've driven Maura crazy with uncertainty about whether I even *know* what's going on. Well, yes, I *think* I do, most of the time, even though I also have that old fear that too much serenity leads not to Nirvana but to the bad kind of stoicism that makes ex-Marines shoot their families.

And I fall victim to my own panic. Last night when I was doing my weekly volunteer hours as an EMT, we transported a woman who had the worst headache of her life and a temperature of 104. At the hospital, while I was giving the nurse the rundown on the woman's symptoms, the nurse interrupted me to ask the woman if she could touch her chin to her chest, which the woman couldn't, because her head hurt so much. "That's not good," I heard the nurse murmur, a comment that made me feel stupid for not having asked the woman to try the same thing (or, for that matter, for not having taken her temperature). Back in the ambulance, I mentioned worriedly to Phil, the paramedic, that the nurse seemed to be suspecting meningitis, and I said it in a way that hinted at my own incompetence for not thinking the same thing.

"I learned a long time ago," said Phil, "that if you hear something with four legs galloping toward you, look for a horse not a zebra."

Meaning, of course, that she probably just had a headache and a fever.

Anyway, we're only halfway through. I wouldn't say it's boring, but only that the pregnancy is just *there*, like a flowerbed. You don't have to pay attention to it all the time. At least I don't. I suppose Maura does, especially since people constantly remind her of it. The fall semester starts tomorrow, and when Maura's been down on campus for preliminary meetings, people have exclaimed, "Whoa! *You've* had a productive summer!" Other people call out across the parking lot, "When are you due?!" She'll be on display when she steps into the classroom again, though she'll probably get a different reaction from most of the students—or none at all. She said that the ones she's run into so far have avoided looking at or mentioning her belly, in the same way a shy man might try to keep his eyes off a woman's prominent cleavage. The efforts at politeness are slapstick comedy.

The tomatoes are ripening like crazy, and for the past week there has been a constantly full bowl of them on the kitchen counter, even though I keep eating from it. It's like that magic bowl of the children's story—put one of anything in (a bean, a gold coin, a cat) and the bowl will produce an endless number of them until you turn the bowl over. Many of the peppers are ready too, and we've also got basil. Italian food is on the menu for the foreseeable future.

AUGUST 25

School has begun again for Maura and me, and Maeve's kindergarten starts next week, after Labor Day. Ever since Maeve was born, the chairs of our departments—here and back in Arkansas—have put Maura and me on opposite schedules, with one of us teaching on MWF and the other on TTh. We can avoid daycare this way, though the downsides are that there isn't a lot of non-Maeve time on our off-days to prepare for class, do research and writing, and grade papers, and that we have to suffer through the assumptions from our parents and nonacademic friends that we don't really work much at all. It's like my friend James wrote in an email at the beginning of the summer, after I had dropped him a note with a description of my garden planting and my relief that school was over: "You people only work 3/4 of the time, and as far as I can see only do 3/4 of the work then." And he used to *be* a professor before he took a 9 to 5 job. "Hey," I told him, "this is why I *went* into academia." It sure wasn't the money.

Maura was hunkered away at the computer all of last evening, and I saw her only at dinner, when she was quiet and distracted. She's got to give a lecture today, and was getting that in shape. She finally put it all aside about ten and came downstairs to say that she'd been depressed all afternoon and evening and had just figured out that it was out of fear that we'd barely see each other for the next three or four months. Each year at this time we pledge to line up babysitters for weekly gigs so we can have a date, and then we don't. We made the same promise last night.

AUGUST 29

The idea of not getting a babysitter suddenly seems nothing more than trivial. In the wake of today's events, which leave me barely able to write, yesterday's relative lack of anxiety is a distant memory. Right now, my mind is spinning and my eyes are watery and my body is filled with sand out to the fingertips. You experience trauma on a big scale—9/11 changing everyone's view of the world—but then it happens on a personal scale and the same kind of seismic shift occurs. Nothing is the same as yesterday.

Maura's mom is on a cruise, from Copenhagen to New York. Earlier this evening, in the middle of the North Atlantic, while sitting on deck and looking at the sun going down over the brilliant fiords and icebergs, she collapsed. Within minutes she was rushed to the ship's infirmary. She went unconscious, stopped breathing. The staff intubated her and put her on a respirator. That's where she is now. They suspect a massive stroke, a brain aneurysm.

Everything we know at this moment, which is not enough, we know because Gail's friend Bill, who is traveling with her, called on the ship's satellite phone. I answered. It was about 8:00. I had been washing dishes. Maura was upstairs checking her email. Bill was gentle, not telling me everything but taking great care to say several times, "This is not trivial." Gail was unconscious, and they were waiting for her to wake up. That would be the best thing, he said, if she woke up. "Okay," I kept saying. "Okay." Maura had come downstairs after she'd heard the urgency in my voice when I called up to ask her whether she knew if her mom was on any medications or had any allergies. These were things the doctors wanted to know. It must've initially confused her to have such questions come out of the blue. But then she was right beside me, in that awful position of having to wait until the other person gets off the phone but knowing you don't want to be there then. "Okay," I said to Bill, trying to collect myself and be ready to turn to Maura and tell her what Bill had told me. He said they were going to watch Gail all night, that he'd call us back in the morning. Each time he spoke, there was a two-second delay, emphasizing just how far away the ship was.

"Okay," I told him. My hands were still damp from the dishwater.

When I spoke to Maura, I felt almost as if my own words would reach her two seconds after my lips moved. I heard myself trying to have the same tone as Bill, though I'd gone numb with fear and I could see the same happening to Maura. Here is that terrible thing, I thought, as I spoke the words. That thing you know but can't believe has been lurking behind you, underneath you, above you forever. I used almost the exact words that Bill had, tried to ease the description onto Maura as he had tried to ease it onto me. I'm not sure I've ever felt such pain, seeing what each word did to her, the word "stroke" bringing a gasp to her face. When I ran out of words, we held each other in front of the sink. Pure contact. There seemed nothing else to do.

And then we had to do something. We got the globe and looked at the North Atlantic, as if that would bring us closer to the ship. Of course it didn't. So I called our friend Lisa, who is an emergency-room nurse, to ask practical questions. "It's not a good sign that she's unconscious," Lisa said. She ran through for me the typical things that happen with stroke victims, and the treatments they usually get. "What kind of medical facilities do they have on the ship?" she asked. I had no idea. What I could imagine was not comforting. What we knew was what Bill had told us: that the ship was off the coast of Greenland — "about as far from anything as it could be" —, that the captain and doctor had decided against getting a helicopter out to evacuate her, because the weather was iffy and the transfer to a helicopter would be too traumatic, and that the captain had ordered full-steam-ahead for the next port with a hospital. That was St. John's, Newfoundland, two days away. "Treatment usually has to happen faster than two days," Lisa said ominously.

Gail is sixty-seven and as healthy as anyone I know. She is only two years into her retirement, traveling, living a glorious life, doing exactly what she wants.

Before bed, I went on-line and found the web site for the cruise line, to see if there was any information about the ship's infirmary. There wasn't. What I did find was a link to a webcam mounted on the bow of the ship. You could get a picture of exactly what the captain might see at that moment, though much grainier. But of course it was still night out there, and the screen was completely black.

AUGUST 30

We slept fitfully, helplessly, and for only a few hours. What little sleep we got was broken up by stretches of ceiling-staring. I got up once to walk the dog. He needed it, but so did I. The feeling of helplessness, of disconnection, had to be countered by fresh night air.

By 9:00 this morning we were able to get the ship's doctor on the phone, only to find out that things had gotten much worse in the night. Bleeding had continued inside Gail's skull, and the doctor was kind but blunt. It was an irreversible coma, he explained, and during the night they had witnessed the classic signs of progressive brain death—seizures, etc. They'd done every clinical diagnostic test they could to assure themselves. "There is nothing to be done," said the doctor. His name is Dr. Bruno Casaregole, he is Italian, and he speaks so gently, but of course his news is shocking and paralyzing. It is almost impossible for me to type these words.

Throughout the day, Maura and Jennifer had to consult by phone — between themselves, with their cousin David who is a doctor in Florida, with the cruise line's medical director in Los Angeles, with Gail's brother in Albany, with the doctor on the ship, with Gail's dear friend Bill who is there with her — and decide whether or not to take their mother off the ventilator. The calls to the ship were unreliable, because the satellite phone was often down. When we did get through, there was that two-second delay.

Maura and Jennifer asked David to call the ship and talk to the doctor himself. He did, then called Maura to say — even more gently than Dr. Casaregole, if that's possible — that he agreed with the diagnosis, with the hopelessness. The conclusion is that the aneurysm was so severe that, as David said, even if she had been standing in the Mayo Clinic when it happened, there would have been nothing they could do for her. It's little solace.

Maeve had a friend over for a play-date all afternoon. It had been arranged beforehand, but we kept it because Maeve needed distraction, and because we were on the phone constantly.

In the afternoon, when she and Jennifer had made their decision, Maura had to write a letter giving Dr. Casaregole permission to unhook the ventilator. It was one paragraph, to the point, full of bravery. She faxed it to the cruise line's medical director in Los Angeles, who had to convince his lawyers that it was sufficient.

I held Maura as much as I could all evening, and she cried, and I cried. It got dark.

And at about ten, the doctor called again. I tried to imagine what he had been going through during the day, and all I could come up with was a picture of him and his staff working quietly, earnestly, with the beep of the heart monitor, the hush of the ventilator. Nothing more specific, and yet the image was almost calming, compared to the intensity of our day.

I listened on the upstairs extension. Dr. Casaregole told Maura that they were prepared. Did she have any requests? Yes, she wanted to be there. But short of that, she wanted to be there through the doctor himself, and I've never heard someone be able to provide such an impossibility so well, so empathetically. They talked, calmly, gently, about temporality, about the land mines we walk across from birth to death, about Gail's spirituality, about the need all of us have for being able to ask so much of others — of strangers — at these moments. To listen to them was a means of decompression for myself, a countershock to the words Bill had spoken the evening before. I felt them right me, as they seemed to be doing for Maura herself. Dr. Casaregole joined Maura in her philosophical wanderings, helped her slow movements toward goodbye, reassured her that he and Bill were standing in for her at Gail's bedside. He described for her the fiords the ship had been passing through in the hours before Gail's stroke, the beauty of the icebergs, the glory of the entire day. "The last things she saw," he said, "were the sights of one of the most pristine places on earth. We all wish for such beautiful final hours."

"Yes, yes," Maura agreed softly.

And when we hung up, we waited in the silence of our own home, with Maeve asleep in her room, the dog pacing, both of us imagining and trying not to imagine the machinery going quiet, the gentle prayers said, Gail's breathing stopping, as the doctor assured us it would, within minutes.

Maura cried heavy and long, and I held her. I felt in shock, and I nodded helplessly as Maura sobbed and gasped for breath.

SEPTEMBER 4

Here in this small town in Vermont, where we arrived yesterday, Maura and Jennifer, both heavily pregnant, walk around and try to let people hug them, though everyone has trouble figuring out how to reach around their bellies. They smile apologetically, and everyone chuckles. These are moments of brief respite from the sadness and disbelief.

I like it better with many people here. I drove over by myself three days ago, to look for Gail's will. The house is so familiar to me, and Gail had left it as clean as if someone might rent it while she was gone, but I couldn't settle in at all. I walked around constantly, with no real plan. On the dining table was a small box with a pair of glass earrings that Gail had bought for my mom and didn't mail before her cruise. On the kitchen counter were a couple notes for errands she'd have to do after she got back. There was unopened mail on the floor underneath the front-door mail slot, and I realized that there was no one to open it but me. I opened the bills, to check due dates. I didn't turn on the TV, didn't cook on the stove, opened the refrigerator only to see if anything needed to be thrown out. Nothing did. I stayed up well past midnight, going idly through file cabinets, through drawers, feeling like an intruder, not knowing exactly what might be worth taking back to Syracuse. I packed up anything of value, to get it out of the house: jewelry, silver, books of photographs. I found a draft of a will, but not a finalized one. And I found a key to a safe-deposit box, where the real will probably was. I slept on the sofa, because I was too uneasy to get under the covers in a bed.

Now, back here again with Maura, Jennifer, Andy, and the kids, we're engaged in the simultaneously consuming activities of grieving and planning a funeral. At least the house has inevitably gotten noisy and messy again, especially with Maeve and Eamon running around. We have to cook meals, make more phone calls, write an obituary, find hotel rooms for people coming to the funeral.

We go constantly all day, with little sleep. I'm getting four hours and then waking up and wondering whether to get up or lie still in the dark and count the minutes. We're each tempted to wallow and let someone else do the work, but it's also a blessing that there is no one else to do the most essential tasks. Who would Maura and Jennifer trust to pick out a casket? To choose the clothes in which their mother will be buried? All four of us need to meet with Gail's lawyer, to find out how we go about dealing with this house. Because we're only here this week, there's a sense of urgency to every task, even the ones that could wait until after the funeral.

The ship will arrive in New York City today, and the funeral director here has driven down to pick up the body.

SEPTEMBER 6

What to say about the funeral? The mass was crowded, hot. All of the family members proceeded in behind the casket. In front were Maura and Jennifer and Sheila, two of them quite pregnant. It was a juxtaposition a heavy-handed movie director would insist upon, but I know that it tore my heart out nonetheless, and probably did the same to most other people in the church. In his eulogy, the priest naturally could not pass up the opportunity to wave his hand toward Maura and Jennifer and talk about how one generation replaces the previous. It was a literary device handed to him on a plate.

Gail was buried next to Maura's father, who died unexpectedly eighteen years ago, when he was only fifty-two. I suppose the imminence of death ought to make any sane person deeply afraid about having a child. We go on only because sanity has nothing to do with it.

SEPTEMBER 9

Today, on my first day back teaching since the funeral, we were talking in my sophomore lit class about Bharati Mukherjee's short story "The Management of Grief." I didn't plan it that way, but I told the students, "You see how literature is so *close* to life sometimes." The story is about several people whose husbands and wives and children died when their plane was blown up on a trans-Atlantic flight—almost, coincidentally, exactly above the route of Gail's cruise ship. The narrator walks through the following months with a valium-induced numbness; another character, a scientist, unsuccessfully tries to find solace in rational thought (it is right that the sharks should eat the bodies, he thinks, because that's what sharks do); and a third person, a woman who has lost her husband and her daughter, joins an ashram in India, eventually claiming to have found serenity through a brief encounter with a young girl who sang and looked exactly like her own daughter. The story is so much about hope. What is its nature? Its purpose? Its possibilities? How do you overcome—or at least accept—such tragedy, such loss? Or why do you *not* accept it? A number of characters in the story never do, but instead live in such denial that they refuse to sign the forms the government requires in order to give them their death benefits. A signature is a giving up of hope. Better to have your electricity turned off, to be evicted from your apartment, to endure your own suffering rather than to deny the slimmest possibilities. No one in the story *manages* grief too well. It is simply too powerful, and it impels characters into journeys both overly rational and irrational, toward little that resembles a new sanity. I don't know how much the students got out of the story. I felt afterwards as if I'd talked myself through it for fifty minutes, as if it were exactly the story I needed.

Maura has been named executor of her mother's estate. Already our lives are filled with the tasks of paying bills, canceling credit cards, consulting with lawyers. Colleagues at work have generously taken over Maura's classes for this week, to give her a little more time off.

SEPTEMBER 10

We had the appointment today for the ultrasound, and I had to force myself to remember that we're having a baby. My mind has been so much elsewhere for the past twelve days. The transition from complete sadness to trying to feel excitement and joy is an incredible wrench.

Nonetheless, the baby continues to grow, seemingly undeterred by the inertia those of us outside the womb currently feel. And so we crowded into the dark room with Tim, the radiologist, and watched him work his way down the image of the baby, beginning at the head and going on to spine, heart, kidneys, bladder. I couldn't help but think of that webcam from Gail's cruise ship, which I had looked at during daylight hours only to find bleak, gray, grainy images of ocean. The resolution on the ultrasound was much sharper.

"Do you want to know now, or do you want me to tell you later?" Tim asked after he'd finished measuring the bladder.

"You're in the area," I said.

"Tell us now," Maura said.

"Well, that there," he said, pointing a little arrow at a distinct shape, "is a penis. An impressively large one, I'd say. And those are the testicles."

There was a momentary silence, which Tim filled by asking, "Is that what you wanted?"

I couldn't think of what to answer. Walking into the clinic, Maura, Maeve, and I had all felt certain it would be a girl. As Maeve had said, "We just know."

When Tim asked his question, Maeve was in the next room watching a video of *Pocahontas*. The receptionist had set her up. Too bad, because she would've handled the moment better than I did. I was sitting behind Tim, and so he couldn't see the way I was *trying* to answer but couldn't think of the right words. What I knew I should do was lean over and kiss Maura joyfully, as I had when we'd found out Maeve was a girl, but the room was small and Tim was in the way. I held onto Maura's foot. She was smiling warily, trying to get a read on my reactions.

Tim kept scanning the rest of the body, and the penis kept floating into view, like a bat circling a streetlight.

"This thing's so big I can hardly see around it," he said, a line with which he undoubtedly flatters every new parent of a boy—but one that probably works every time.

"We're surprised it's a boy," I finally managed to admit, "but we're not surprised by how *much* of a boy it is."

That broke the momentary tension. Still, as Tim kept giving the kid the once over, measuring the long bones, counting the number of toes and fingers, looking at the shape of the spinal column, making sure there were two kidneys and two lungs, I sat back in my chair and thought of that scene in *Butch Cassidy and the Sundance Kid* when the two of them jump off the cliff.

Maura was looking at me with a wary smile, and I tried to smile heartily back. But she could see that I was dumbfounded. Anyway, is my mind to be trusted? It feels too shocked by this series of surprises. All I could really tell her, after we'd stumbled out of the office and were driving to get a celebratory milk shake, was that I can't absorb any more news. All I want from here on are things that I expect. I need to sleep on this.

By the way, every other part of the kid's body looks healthy. In all the craziness of the last weeks, I actually forgot that they might not be.

It undoubtedly sounds weird and small-minded to say that it's hard for me to think of myself as a man who has a son, but it's true so far. It was easier to tell Maeve that she'll be having a brother. There's a word that's easier for me to comprehend, partly because I have two of them and partly because the word has other connotations: caretaker, pal. A son is something to control. This fear got reinforced right away, in the ultrasound room itself, as the radiologist — one of the nicest guys I've run into lately, a guy who seems gentle and humane and full of good humor — told us that he was the wildest of boys, that his parents kept shaking their heads all through his childhood and saying "If you make it to kindergarten" and then "If you make it to high school" and finally "If you make it to adulthood it'll be a miracle."

It's hard to tell what Maeve thinks. Earlier today she wanted a sister, the worries about having to share her dresses seemingly abated. At the end of the ultrasound, before Tim turned off his machinery, I'd called her in to let her see the image on the screen. She hadn't wanted to leave the movie. Pocahontas and John Smith were falling in love. But she came in, absorbed the news, told me politely that she hadn't *really* wanted only a sister, and then insisted on going right back to the TV room. Afterwards, she was a bit whiny, but probably more from tiredness and disappointment that the video was over than from the fact that she wasn't getting a sister. But who knows? We'll try to get a read on it over the next day or two.

I'm so far behind already in my work for school. I went heavy on the reading and writing assignments this semester, and for the past ten days I haven't opened a book.

SEPTEMBER 11

It's the next morning, and I had another football dream. This time, I was standing in the backyard with a white football that fit comfortably and softly into my hands. I was waiting for someone to throw it to, and there was no danger of painful contact. I suppose this is a trite and obvious but promising sign.

We won't be able to name him Abigail.

SEPTEMBER 12

This morning at the bus stop, we told Lynniece that we were having a boy. Lynniece is the mother of Maeve's best friend, Curtis, who is six.

Lynniece was holding her infant daughter Emily to her breast, feeding her in the morning sun, a pink blanket draped over the baby's head. Lynniece immediately burst out laughing. The laughter seemed an involuntary response, and of course I told her how much it comforted me, just as much as did the subsequent stories about her brother and his string of accidents as he was growing up, including the time he caught himself on fire.

She said that when Curtis was born she had no idea what to do with this "thing," since there had been so many girls in her family. "But they're really sweet," she insisted once she got her laughter under control. "You don't think they will be, but they surprise you. It's like you're yelling and laughing all the time." And then she laughed again and wished us good luck.

SEPTEMBER 13

Maeve has been asking Maura: "If you die, who will take care of me and the baby?" Of course Maura assures her that no one is going to die for a long, long time, that Maeve will be very, very old — at least thirty or forty — before Maura dies. She reminded her that Gail's mother was only five days short of a hundred when she died ("One hundred!" Maeve exclaimed), and that by that time Gail was already a grandmother — evidence to counter the recent scary events.

"I don't want her to be too worried about our dying," Maura told me later.

I said that it seems too early to know where this new knowledge might lodge into her subconscious, what effect it might have — and that all we can do is talk with her about it, give her a sense of security. And not die.

"She was very generous," Maura said. "She said, 'If you die, Mommy, I'll take care of the baby.'"

SEPTEMBER 14

Last night I got up to take the dog for what seemed a necessary walk at 1:30, and then soon after I crawled into Maeve's single bed with her because she'd woken up and said she was scared of the dark. It took her about an hour of worming around before she fell back asleep. The only thing missing that would've made the night well-rounded was changing a couple of diapers. And that's right around the corner. I can barely wake up this morning. Again, I think this is all nuts.

The dog threw up this morning in Maeve's room and was stumbling around. I was upstairs and Maura called me for help. The dog seemed okay when I got there, though, and I took him for a slow walk around the block. He's so old that I have trouble imagining how he's going to make it to the winter, much less *through* it.

Actually, I fear that he and the baby are on converging paths, the dog going toward death and the baby toward birth, and that they'll reach their respective destinations at exactly the same moment, on a snowy and undriveable day in early January. That would be par for the course.

SEPTEMBER 15

The idea of a boy is slowly taking hold, I guess. Maura immediately switched from calling it *her* to calling it *him*, and I asked with wonder how she could do that so easily. "I'm still getting used to it," she claimed, but the hesitation doesn't show through.

Jennifer thinks it's great news.

My brother Steve laughed over the phone from Los Angeles and loved imagining how I'll deal with the kid when he's fifteen and starts getting into the kind of crap Steve put my parents through at that age.

"Seriously, though, this baby will fill your heart with love," Steve told Maura. "It'll make up in some way for your mother's death."

I told our friend Mike, father of the immeasurably cute three-year-old Willie. He admitted that the presence of those two older sisters has mostly squashed any boyish troublemaking in Willie. "But last week," Mike said, "Willie spent an hour or so in his room with one of his friends, and when he came out I saw this glint in his eye, as if he'd discovered something in there with another boy that was liberating." Mike laughed, and I heard in it a little of my own trepidation.

I told our friend Bill, the man who was on the ship with Gail, that the baby's a boy. He doesn't have any children himself, but he's got several brothers, and he immediately understood my wariness. "Well," he said with the wisdom that comes from a deep acceptance of the way the world is, "other people have done it. Other people of less intelligence, less height, less humor, less shoe size. That's about all the comfort you can probably have."

Strangely, his words gave me about the most comfort I've felt in a long time.

SEPTEMBER 16

In one of my classes we're reading Gretel Ehrlich's *The Solace of Open Spaces*, a beautiful book that Ehrlich wrote out of the death of her lover and her subsequent move to Wyoming to let the land heal her—a process that took years. It's the sixth or seventh time I've read the book, and it's the first time the undercurrent of grief has seemed to color everything else in the book for me. I don't know how I'll ask my students to talk about it. It's a book I want to keep to myself, to let flow over me and give silent articulation to my own sorrows.

Maura is back teaching and is taking her students through a different kind of story: the fourteenth-century *Sir Gawain and the Green Knight*. The poem is full of impending doom—Gawain is required to fight the much more powerful Green Knight and fully expects to have his head chopped off—but in the days before that everyone at court is trying to distract Gawain, trying to get him to have some fun, even while they are sad at heart themselves. One woman, for example, repeatedly tries to seduce him. Lust is not on Gawain's mind, but the temptress does arouse in him an erotic desire for life and joy. And so the story, Maura tells her students, is not about the test of Gawain's virtue and fortitude—both qualities he does possess—but about joy in the face of deathly fear and sadness.

"I tell them," Maura said to me, "that joy is a virtue. God wants you to have it, but sometimes you have to work for it when you don't feel like it."

"Kind of like right now?" I asked.

"Yes," she said. "Kind of like right now."

SEPTEMBER 18

How quickly the comfort of this pregnancy dissipates. Now we're barreling through rapids again, holding our oars tightly, cold water spraying over us. This morning Maura had her monthly checkup with her OB. He hadn't yet received the report from the ultrasound lab, and so we waited in the exam room for a half hour while the report got faxed over. He came back in and said, ever so casually, "Did they tell you about this funny little thing in his heart?"

Pause. "No."

He explained. Something called "echogenic cardiac focus." A white spot on the ultrasound that may indicate some abnormality of the pappilary muscles inside the chambers of the heart. I thought I was pretty much to the point of numbness, but having a doctor tell you that there may be heart abnormalities in your baby is a reliable way to get a response. So is the fact that an echogenic cardiac focus is one of the markers they look for as a sign for possible Down syndrome. But if it's the only marker present—no abnormally short thigh bones, no abnormal slanting of the forehead—then it probably doesn't mean anything. Probably.

"In the vast majority of these cases," the doctor said, "these things disappear by the time you have the next ultrasound. They seem to resolve themselves. So we're going to schedule you for another ultrasound in four weeks."

Maura and I nodded, not asking him what happens if this thing doesn't resolve itself. The question entered my head, but I couldn't imagine it being healthy to speak it in the tension of that small room. It would have sounded like a gunshot.

"You didn't need another thing thrown at you right now, did you?" he asked Maura. She had told him earlier about her mother dying.

She smiled and through a trembling lip whispered, "No."

SEPTEMBER 19

The bane of technology is that if you only want to know the sex, you get reams of other information that you don't want. Before an echogenic cardiac focus ever showed up on an ultrasound in 1987 (I immediately fought technology with technology by going on the web to get *more* information), these things resolved themselves in the dark of the fetus's body without anyone ever knowing about it. I hate to be a Luddite and say we were better off that way, but right now I feel we were better off that way. And I only say that because what I did find on the web backed up Maura's doctor's optimism. Most sites that looked reliable said that while these "bright spots" have been showing up more frequently on ultrasounds in the second trimester—technicians seem to be finding them like astronomers find new supernovas—most experts agree that having one doesn't mean your heart will pump blood as efficiently as a chewed-up rubber dog toy or that you need to dig through the filing cabinets right now to make sure your insurance covers open-heart surgery. What having one *does* mean, I don't know.

Just before the doctor gave us this news, Maura and I had been sitting politely in the exam room ignoring the stack of parenting magazines and talking about control—as in the fact that we have about as much of it right now as we have sleep. Maura was saying—more to herself, I think—that we needed to just let things happen as they may, to be centered in the present and not waste energy living in fear or frustration. I think she was thinking about Perry, who died despite Maura's attempts to give him a good indoor life, and of course about her mother. But that has its limits, as she pointed out. "I can't very well tell my students that I'm just going to let things happen, can I?" Maura said.

And then the doctor came in, and there was nothing to do but let things happen.

And then that evening right before dinner, when Maeve was supposed to arrive home from her friend Lainie's, the people who arrived instead were Lainie's mom and dad, who were scouring the neighborhood to *find* Maeve and Lainie.

"They asked if we could walk Maeve home instead of drive, and I said sure," Anne said, "never dreaming they'd begin walking on their own. I called and called, and I couldn't find them anywhere."

Lainie's dad, Jim, took the car and went in one direction. Anne and I went on foot, splitting up at the corner to cover both sides of the blocks. I was running in my flip-flops, which kept sliding off. Lainie lives four blocks away, and on my whole way there I kept yelling "Fuck" and then muttering about how Maeve *knows* not to cross the street alone, and that she simply wouldn't have disappeared like this.

Anne and I reached her house at the same time, and Maeve and Lainie were in the backyard, being taken care of by a neighbor, whom Lainie had sought out when she and Maeve realized that no one else was in the house. They'd been hiding under a bed on the third floor, and insisted they hadn't heard Anne yelling. Anne and I both tried not to yell right then.

I walked Maeve home.

"I was never hurt," Maeve explained with a confidence that I tried to temper without crushing. And it's true that she *hadn't* been in danger. And it was the adults who were the ones who needed to chill out. Nonetheless, by the time we got home, she understood what would happen if she ever pulled a trick like that again.

SEPTEMBER 22

I give the baby a new name each day. "How's Hector?" I ask Maura. Or "How's Abdul?" "Did Nils sleep through the night?" "What's Jack got to say for himself today?" But they're all just jokes, meant to stave off the feeling that time is going by quickly and no magic is occurring in the naming biz.

Maura was sitting in the digesting chair last night after dinner and mentioned that within a week or two she'll be entering her third trimester. I didn't believe her. Most of the time lately I haven't remembered what month it is.

"October, November, December," she counted out on her fingers.

"Slow it *down*," I urged.

I remember that at about this time with the Maeve pregnancy, we were lolling about like Paul Newman and Joanne Woodward in *The Long, Hot Summer*, trying to come up with things to occupy us while Maeve simmered slowly and gained those few extra pounds.

Today Maura got a letter from her friend Cindy, down in Annapolis, who wrote about how Hurricane Isabel flooded their downtown but that they were, fortunately, high and dry. "I hope that you have not been too distraught or distracted to enjoy your pregnancy," Cindy wrote. "Are you not in that particularly invigorating trimester?"

SEPTEMBER 23

We've gotten a routine down with the dog, in which he'll get up and pace during the night for an hour or two, and in the morning, Maura, bleary-eyed and pissed off, will say to him, "You're on the short road to euthanasia."

SEPTEMBER 24

This morning in the paper there was an article about a 15-year-old boy who has been suspended for two weeks for spraying "Fart Spray" in the hallway at school, and I showed it to Maura and said, "Here is our future."

SEPTEMBER 25

Here's an insight: A pregnancy is never about the father. I say this with only a little resentment. What I actually feel more of is befuddlement. It truly does surprise me, in the same way I've been surprised that people's generous reactions to Gail's death — condolences, invitations to coffee or lunch, hugs — have almost all been directed at Maura, even though it was also my mother-in-law who died. I can't begin to imagine what Maura's grief is really like. It must be exponentially more than mine. Still, all of these reactions have occasionally made me wonder whether I really did have anything of a close relationship with Gail.

Maura is the only one who's recognized this odd discrepancy. "You should go out and talk with people, take your own time to relax," she says. And I tell her that no one has yet called with an invitation. Then she says that tomorrow morning she has to leave early because someone wants to buy her breakfast.

I got an email today from a friend of mine back in Arkansas. Here's the total content of her message: "How's Maura?"

And so it goes.

I'm thinking about all this today because Jennifer and Andy's baby is due in a week and a half, and I had a long talk on the phone with Jennifer yesterday about how Andy for the last few days has been wondering aloud what his job is, and why he might be needed. The catalyst was that a couple of weeks ago they hired a doula, a woman whose job is to help the mother through labor, and this seems to have made Andy feel that he might as well stay home and watch the Packers instead of being in the delivery room. It didn't help that the doula basically ignored his presence altogether. I have almost complete sympathy for his desire to be useful. Still, I can understand why he said "I don't know" when Jennifer asked him, "If I told you that what I really want you to do is to be there to say you love me, would you believe me?"

When I reported this to Maura later (there are few secrets among the four of us), she got riled up and said, "See, this is just the thing a woman understands and most men don't."

"What?" I said.

"That it's enough to be there to say he loves her. That that's *important.*"

"He'll come around," I said. "He's just working through it. This is not a piece of cake for the father."

I appreciated that she didn't disagree.

"He'll come around," I said again. And in fact later that evening Jennifer called to say, with a lot of relief in her voice, that Andy *had* arrived home earlier with a healthier attitude, apologizing for "venting."

Maura's toying with the idea of getting her own doula, and even asked her OB at her last appointment whether he'd mind. He wouldn't. I haven't said so to her yet, but I'm against it. We got along perfectly fine last time, and I can't fathom any difference now. Then it occurs to me that Maura may want to hire someone as a mother-replacement. The thought makes me uneasy.

SEPTEMBER 26

Ever since Perry died, the neighborhood bully cats have been wandering into our backyard, sensing that this is now territory free for the taking. Lila is too meek to scare them off.

"What we need is a dog," Maura said. "Unfortunately, all we've got is Calvin."

It's unfortunate for Lila, who got chased up onto the back steps and trapped against the screen door one evening earlier this week. I had to run out and rescue her, but for days after that she wouldn't go outside. She slept in the closet upstairs. Then we noticed an abscess on her back just in front of her tail, and so yesterday she went to the vet to get that drained. Now she's asleep in her cat bed, shaved from the midsection to her tail, with tubes in her to let the pus drain. She obviously doesn't like this new arrangement any more than the rest of us.

Poor kitty.

SEPTEMBER 27

Next morning's news flash: Jennifer's water broke last night. They're on the short road to an early delivery.

Saturday evening: Jennifer called. They went ahead with a C-section, because there was no significant labor action. Baby's out and healthy. Jennifer's fine. The girl is seven pounds, six ounces, and nineteen inches long. She's ten days early. They've named her Neve Abigail.

Andy's fine. Turns out he didn't have to get into a shoving match with the doula after all. Jennifer canned the doula at the last minute, when it became clear that there would be no natural childbirth, and when a couple of close friends showed up to be with her in the recovery room.

We're helping to make calls to relatives, tell them the news. I imagine that Gail knows.

OCTOBER 1

First frost last night, and there were even snowflakes twirling in the breeze yesterday, at the same time that there was a glorious rainbow. From the hill where I studied it, the feet of the rainbow rose thickly and with rich colors. The middle of the arc was missing—invisible in the clouds—but the feet were specifically planted, one by the fire station, the other by the tire shop over on Erie Boulevard, places I drive by frequently, touched for these moments by something magical that the people on the scene couldn't know about.

OCTOBER 2

I think more and more about not teaching anymore after this year, and just staying home to take care of the kids. I imagine, sometimes, how satisfying and healthy it would be to homeschool Maeve, even if we do happen to be in one of the best public school districts in New York, and even if there are other good—if overly expensive—choices, as well: the Catholic school, a top-notch private school. Despite all these schools' high ratings, I have all kinds of hesitations about how Maeve is going to be corrupted and dumbed down and have her creativity and patience squashed by being in *any* school—with its schedules designed to allow the efficient herding of kids from music to recess, from art to snack time. I'm diligently trying to be patient about how much her kindergarten class is concentrating on recognizing the letters in their names, when in fact she's been able to spell her name for three years now. I try not to say aloud, Couldn't we pick up the pace a little?

On the other hand, yesterday when she got home from school, she began sounding out words. It was a game she started herself, and she asked me to give her words to read. So I printed them out one-by-one on an index card, and she read each one: *blob, bedroom, video, grass, glass, stapler, desk, swan, tooth.* . . . With only a little help now and then, she got each one, usually within a couple seconds. My guess is that we're on that cusp of literacy. Everyone says that once a kid is ready, it happens fast. Perhaps kindergarten has brought it on. Perhaps it would've happened anyway.

On the good side, last week her homework was to fill out a "Responsibility Sheet" each night — and so we had some leverage to get her to clear her plate after dinner or help make her bed or something else that's often not worth the battle.

Before she started kindergarten, I'd never heard the word "bored" come from Maeve's mouth, and suddenly this is one of her lines. She already intones it like a fifteen-year-old. Grocery shopping is boring. Playing in the backyard is boring. She's likely to be bored forever if she can't watch a video right when she gets home from school. Sorry, I say, no videos until after you eat lunch and play outside and do some other healthier things. And maybe not then. I'm a monster with the videos. Of course she whines and cries about imminent insanity and the frustrations of being a kid, but these last only three or four minutes. Then she's immersed in playing with dolls or coloring. One afternoon last week, we went through the brief battle, which she lost, and then she colored for three hours straight, stopping only to take sips from the juice or munch on the snacks I'd occasionally place by her elbow.

Anyway, she's also using the word sloppily. She claimed yesterday that she was bored with going to the library at school. They go every four days. I couldn't imagine why, since we've so far been able to convince her that libraries are places any sane person would choose over, say, video arcades. When she didn't know video arcades existed, this was an easy and consistently successful argument to make. But now when we go to the mall she sees the arcade, hears its annoying cacophony, and tries to drag me into its evil darkness. I say no, and explain that the noise gives me a headache, which is true but also not *so* true that I don't feel as if I'm lying to her. Fortunately, the health of her father still concerns her, and so she's never actually been in an arcade. If there's time after those mall trips, I take her to the library on the way home for psychological reinforcement. "I have too much trouble deciding on a book," she explained about her boredom with the library at school. But that day she'd picked out a wonderful book, *The Great Quillow* by James Thurber, a book with captivating drawings and lots and lots of words, one that we spent a good half hour reading when she got home. She's not *bored*. She's frustrated. She doesn't get to spend *enough* time in the library. They go for only thirty minutes, and what she really wants—just like when we're at the public library—is to take her damn time.

I'm all for it, though I'm the one rushing her every morning to get up, get dressed, eat something for god's sake, brush your teeth we're already late for the bus and it'll be lucky if you even get to go to school today.

She's learned the value of weekends. On weekends she gets to have what we call "Jane Smiley Time." Smiley's a novelist who wrote an essay once about being allowed to spend all of her Saturday mornings in her room, playing games, taking her dolls through their dramas, daydreaming. She never had to help clean the house during that time or be somewhere else. It's what made her a writer, she said.

We've got a wonderful routine now of waiting for the school bus in the morning. If I ever decide to homeschool Maeve it will take all my willpower to give up these ten minutes of standing at the end of the block with eight or nine kids and three or four other parents, comparing sleeps, catching up on neighborhood gossip, connecting before going our own ways.

OCTOBER 3

I woke up this morning certain of what I wanted to name the baby. When I told it to Maura, she didn't comment on the name, only observed, "It's not a bad thing to wake up in the morning certain of something."

Nights have been rough for Maura lately. As she told Lynniece at the bus stop this morning, if it's not the dog keeping her awake, it's not being able to get comfortable with the big belly, or it's grieving for her dead mother, or it's allergies. "It can be all *kinds* of things," Maura laughed. Her allergies are bad this fall, and she's often awake sneezing, which gives her time to have dark thoughts.

Two nights ago she woke me up at 3:45. She'd been awake since 2:00, sneezing. By the time she woke me up, she was only crying. Groggily, I held her. I let her talk.

"I don't want to have to be okay," she said, between sobs. "I will be okay, sometimes, but I don't want to have to be. But I don't know how I'm supposed to do that. I can't very well break out sobbing in the hallways at school. And every morning I wake up to people I have to take care of," she explained. "Maeve. My students. The estate. Myself. You. The one person whose job it's supposed to be to take complete care of me isn't here. I'm not okay, and I want my mom. I want my mom."

I can't pretend to know how hard it all is for Maura. I do what I can to make things easier—cooking, getting Maeve off to school in the morning. I mopped the entire house this weekend, dusted under the bed and behind the dressers, trying to get out all the dog hair and whatever else is going up Maura's nose at night. It's all small stuff. The other night when she was crying, I held her, told her I was here for whatever she needs.

"That makes it all bearable," she whispered.

This must be what she meant last week when she said that Andy just had to say to Jennifer that he loved her.

OCTOBER 4

Maura made two sugar-free pumpkin pies today. Not for health reasons. She simply forgot the sugar, which we didn't know until we sat down eagerly to toss ourselves into fall cuisine.

"I'm in no shape to be baking," she said.

"Did you know that you used two pie shells for each pie?" I asked. Four pie shells came in the package, but she separated the stack only into two.

"No wonder it's so soggy on the bottom," she said.

The pies went sadly into the garbage.

OCTOBER 5

Bonnie from Bulgaria called today, and because she has a boy, she checked in with how I'm getting used to the idea of my own son.

"Well, it's getting better," I admitted, not wanting to seem as if I'd come on board totally. Actually, the evening before I'd watched a *60 Minutes* segment about the old story of girl fetuses being aborted at such a high rate in India that there was concern over how the future imbalance—not enough wives to be had—would lead anxious men to start wars and cause general mayhem. I was feeling defensive for girls, and not very patient with the men of the world.

"It's like your hair growing," Bonnie assured me. "It's not like they show up one day and are boys. They reveal themselves to you day by day, and even though you might have initially thought you couldn't handle a boy, you do just the same as you handle a girl. Besides, they only want the same thing girls want: to be loved."

"Hair growing. Day by day," I repeated back to her. "I'm writing this down."

OCTOBER 7

To add to the stress of our lives, the Red Sox are in the playoffs. Both Maura and I have been Red Sox fans for life—she because she grew up in New England, and I because I inherited the loyalty from my dad, who never should have had it because he grew up near Cleveland, but he had it anyway.

Maura's the worst Red Sox fan in the world, or maybe the best, depending on how you look at it. She cares for them but can't watch them, like a mother whose daughter is a cliff diver. When the Sox are on TV, she has to cover her eyes or leave the room. I can't even *mention* the 1986 Red Sox loss in the World Series without her nearly going into hyperventilation.

It was a rough weekend. The Sox had to play the Oakland A's in a five-game series, and they lost the first two, nearly fulfilling Maura's pessimistic expectations of them. But then they came back and won the last three, but only barely.

Last night after Maeve was in bed Maura and I sat at the kitchen table, grading papers with the game on the radio low in the background. We pumped our fists and probably got overly generous toward bad student writing when the Red Sox scored, then got depressed and pissed off at one too many comma splices when the A's scored. When it got to the bottom of the ninth and the Red Sox were up 4–3 and the A's started putting men on base, Maura said, "I'm going to bed. Come in and tell me after." I got up from the table and stood over the radio, my shoulders tensed, my arms shaking, while the A's loaded the bases with one out and needed only one hit to win. Then Derek Lowe struck out two batters to avoid the tragedy. I felt as if I might hyperventilate.

I think Maura's afraid that too much Red Sox stress will send her into early labor. What's coming next — a best-of-seven series against the Yankees — just might.

OCTOBER 11

We're in Vermont for the weekend, cleaning out closets and drawers. This is satisfying in a work-ethic kind of way, but it ranks low on the fun-scale otherwise. Maura's been tackling the closets, and I've left her to it as a meditative and prayerful task. When I go up to check on her every couple of hours, she's got another big black plastic bag filled with things to give away, and sometimes her eyes are red from crying. I'll haul the bags over to the Episcopal Church when she's done. I've been working in other rooms, boxing up china and the best pots and pans, recycling old paperwork like every cancelled check that Maura's parents wrote since 1965. Gail was an organized person.

It's unnerving to be stripping the house of signs of her presence. Taking photos from the walls. Wrapping in newspaper the various pieces of pottery that have sat for years on her kitchen counters. Untaping from the refrigerator door her list of items to remember to take with her on her cruises. Every object — and there are so many of them — connotes these heart-stopping memories, and it's easy to see why someone might stand in the middle of the kitchen for fifteen or twenty minutes completely unable to decide whether it's okay to throw away the old mop that the dead person had used. After the funeral, one of Maura's older cousins pulled me out of Maura's hearing range and gave me some advice: "Get Mom back to Syracuse as quickly as possible." He meant to take the pictures and hang them on our walls, to bring back her coffee mugs and drink from them, to give her houseplants a new home on our windowsills. And we had left Vermont that time with a car packed to the gills ("Never leave without a full car" was the cousin's other piece of advice), and I hung pictures right away, found a sunny spot for the plants, gave some of our own coffee mugs to the Salvation Army so we'd have room for Gail's. Maura had her mom's engagement ring resized and is wearing it. It's all helped.

Still, the task of changing this house in Vermont from Gail's house into merely *a* house is painful, especially when we're in its rooms, resting on its familiar furniture, cooking on its familiar stove. It'll be easier when we get back to Syracuse again with another full car.

Perhaps the worst part of it is that we're undoing the very place that Maeve knows so well as her grandmother's house. She calls it "the house that smells good," indicating that her attachments to it are already deep and physical.

Our goal is to get Gail's part of the house in shape to rent, and then hope we can get someone in it over the winter. (The house is split into three apartments, and there are tenants in the other two. As executor of the estate, Maura has suddenly found herself as a long-distance landlord.) I don't think it'll be until next spring that Maura and Jennifer decide whether they want to sell the place or hold onto it for sentimental and investment reasons. This weekend, Maura and I keep trying to imagine why we might make the five-hour trip back to this little town, if we happen to keep at least part of the house open for ourselves. There's the postcard beauty, like this weekend when the leaves are in full color. And there's skiing nearby, though it's probably not fair to put that in the pro column since neither of us actually skis. There's the idyllic comfort of the place, a substantial check in its favor. The house is in the center of town, with the library and the general store right down the street, the park a block in the other direction, the covered bridge across the street, church steeples peeping up on the little skyline. It's a movie-set kind of place, a magic kingdom, as Maura has always referred to Vermont, with a mixture of intense love and eye-rolling. The place is certainly not overly wholesome, since most of the town that Maura grew up in is now owned by zillionaires from Connecticut and Massachusetts who need second homes with forty-seven rooms and little plaques on the front that say "Built in 1788." That's a drawback. (Maura's parents bought their house dirt-cheap in 1970, before the rush.) Anyway, it is "home" for Maura, and the best reason either of us could come up with over the weekend for keeping the house was to keep a connection to that home, and to pass it on to our kids. "To let them know where I'm from," Maura explained.

That's a valid reason. Whether it balances out against the expense and hassle is still up in the air.

OCTOBER 12

Now it's our last full day in Vermont for this trip, and we swore we'd quit cleaning at noon, no matter what condition the place was in, and take Maeve to the park for a picnic. It was bright but slightly chilly, a glorious fall day, and we first sat at a table and ate the Italian grinders we'd gotten from the butcher shop. Then Maeve and I made a big pile of leaves and jumped in them a few times before we had to begin dumping handfuls of them on Maura as she tried to relax under a tree. When I plopped down next to Maura, both of us picking leaf remnants off ourselves, I felt the pull of the season, the nostalgia of my childhood. "I wish I had a son to toss a football with," I admitted.

She laughed. "Maeve can throw a football pretty well," she said.

"But she won't."

"True."

When Maeve ran over to throw more leaves on us, I asked her whether she ever wanted to play soccer. There were kids playing fifty feet away.

"No," she said, then laughed as she tried to stuff leaves down the back of my shirt. "It's boring."

"How about baseball?" I asked.

She didn't answer, just ran off to kick leaves.

"She's got no interest in sports," I said.

OCTOBER 17

I'm not sure what to expect from autumn anymore. It used to be my favorite season — the onset of cold weather, the excavating of winter clothes from the attic — but this is the third fall in a row that has been colored in darker ways than the yellows and reds and oranges. (Two years ago was 9/11. Last year were the miscarriages, the death of a close friend, and the death, in a car accident, of Maeve's preschool teacher.)

The Red Sox have lost. Not without the greatest of battles, taking the Yankees to seven games and losing in the eleventh inning of the last game. Maura and I sat at the kitchen table until after midnight listening to it, hoping, in joy and then despair, finally exhausted but not able to sleep well. Maura kept waking up all night thinking of the Red Sox. I dreamt that the bathroom sink and counter were falling through a huge crack in the bedroom ceiling—"a dream about collapse," I told Maura.

I'd forgotten the isolation that pregnancy brings. Like birds sitting on a nest, Maura and I are turning more and more inward. Our eyes gravitate toward her belly, and so do our consciousnesses. When Maura was pregnant with Maeve, we hardly saw anyone for the last month or two—or at least rarely wanted to. Now that nesting instinct is emerging again, and we're less inclined to pick up the phone and call anyone, less interested in getting a babysitter and going out. There's a new couple at work whom we've been meaning to invite over for dinner for two months now, but haven't because of the chaos and may very well not now because of the bubble thickening around us.

I don't know if Maeve is feeling this same thing. Going into a bubble has to be harder for the child already present, because it's not in a child's nature to wait quietly, to go interior. When that happens, we usually worry. We think depression or autism.

Yet Maeve has her moments, her reflections, about both death and birth. When we were in Vermont last weekend, she was left alone for a few minutes with Bill, Gail's friend who was with her when she died. I overheard their conversation from the hallway.

"Grandma Gail died because her brain stopped working," Maeve explained to Bill.

"Yes, yes it did," he said.

"I miss her," Maeve said.

"I miss her too," said Bill. "She was a wonderful person. I'm very sad she's not here."

"I'm sad too," Maeve said. "I miss her because she was my grandma."

"Yes, she was," said Bill.

"My cat Perry died, too," Maeve told him. "And my friend Curtis's mouse. I bet Grandma Gail is petting Perry right now, and Perry is chasing Curtis's mouse."

"It sounds like that would make them all happy," Bill said, "except the mouse."

Other times, Maeve will cuddle up next to Maura's belly and talk soothingly to the baby, promising him she'll have sunglasses ready when he comes out because it'll be so bright.

"Day to day remind yourself that you are going to die." That Kathleen Norris quote from Benedict in her book *Dakota* is *still* rattling around in my head and when I thought of it again last night I wondered briefly—and I hoped not improperly—whether perhaps Gail and Perry and Curtis's mouse are all doing their parts to help this pregnancy along, to remind all of us to live properly, as full of awareness as a mouse being chased.

OCTOBER 18

We've gone back for the follow-up ultrasound. The kid is two-and-a-half pounds, and all's well except that funny little thing is still in his heart. It looks like a spot you'd want a photographer to airbrush out. "If I saw this on an ultrasound of my kid," said Tim the technician, "I wouldn't think twice about it." The staff doctor said the same when she took a peek. "Somebody began seeing this and wrote a paper on it," she lamented, "and now we all have to look for it. It's probably been there on many, many fetuses, and no one ever knew it, and there were never any problems. Don't let it concern you."

We came away trusting the both of them and simultaneously certain that, simply to make us feel good, they were lying.

OCTOBER 19

Basic training today. Curtis was over for a couple of hours of playtime. As much as I love Curtis, he only reminded me, as I kept lecturing too loudly to him about not touching this or being careful climbing to the top of that, that my transformation to father-of-a-son is not complete. I see these fathers of sons—like Curtis's dad, Tim—and I think that they have learned some inner peacefulness that will never, ever come to me. Other times I suspect it's simply a willful blindness. Whatever works.

Against all odds, we finally had the new couple from work over for dinner last night. They seemed happy to get out, not only because they're new in town but also because they have a four-month-old boy. If the nesting impulse feels fresh to us, it seems to be getting old for them. They brought the kid with them, and he's quiet and gurgly. I could live with one like that. Maeve, who was relieved to have company, was chattering all evening, occasionally breaking into "This Land is Your Land," and Erin and Miles, who are so awed by the immediate experience of being with their tiny baby, said it was impossible for them to imagine that someday he would actually be talking to them, telling them the foods he likes (or, if he's like Maeve, doesn't like), belting out his own patriotic songs. I remember that inability to imagine beyond the present. I'm feeling it now, but with scarier results. It's *me* I can't imagine growing into something other than what I am at this very instant. I often think, Okay, it's easy to be a decent dad once. The real test is whether you can pull it off the second time around, whether you can avoid gliding. That's one reason I was so much hoping for another girl—so I *could* be the same dad again. Talk about your naïve hopes, your willful blindness.

OCTOBER 20

Not that I need or am collecting additional evidence about boys' antics, but they keep coming, like the story Miles told us about when he and his brother were seven and eight and would pull the control knob off their old TV console to expose an electric coil, onto which they'd put their tongues so that they could be thrown halfway across the room in backwards somersaults.

"You really can't kid-proof your house against idiots like that," he admitted.

OCTOBER 21

I put my foot in my mouth last night by telling Maura that her mind is not working all that well these days. I didn't think I was telling her anything she didn't already know, and she even brought up the subject in the first place. I was simply agreeing and elaborating—attributing it to the pregnancy, which in my mind was a way to *deflect* her self-criticism. I tried to make her laugh by reminding her that after dinner I'd asked her to put the kettle on to boil for some coffee, and she'd filled the kettle and put it on the stove but forgot to turn on the burner. I discovered it ten minutes later when I went into the kitchen to figure out why I wasn't hearing any whistle. My good intentions didn't matter. She got offended.

Then late this morning the dog peed on the carpet in the living room. I had left the house early, and Maura was supposed to be in charge.

"Did you not let the dog out this morning?" I asked her when I got home, after I cleaned up and let the dog out.

She hadn't. It was beyond me to figure out how someone could not remember to let the dog out. Of course, she probably would have had to carry him down the stairs.

"Are you mad at me?" she asked after a significant pause.

"Not mad," I said, really trying not to sound as mad as I was. "I'm a little annoyed."

Really, what I wanted to say was that I don't mind taking up a lot of the slack during this pregnancy, but that there are some basic things I wouldn't expect to *have* to do. And, to be really honest, that today I'm feeling a bit tired of taking care of everything, of Maura having excuses out the wazoo. The pregnancy. The dead mother. The inability to sleep. Yada yada. This morning she was up at five, and I found her sitting largely and uncomfortably in the digesting chair, grading papers, when I got up at seven. She was in a lousy mood all day. I kept wanting to ask her, the way Maeve's preschool teacher used to ask her, "Is there a smile in your pocket?" There was more likely a rock in Maura's pocket that she'd heave at me.

Cripes. It was a lousy day. It didn't help when she apologized and finally told me that she'd felt crappy all day: sore throat, sinus headache, and chills.

I plow along, foot deeper in mouth.

OCTOBER 22

Tonight for dinner Maura made a chili by throwing together some things from cans, and I told her it tasted kind of like college food, in a good way. She seemed to like the comment. We each had a helping, then she went to the stove and brought the pan back. There was only one more helping.

"Is it okay with you if I finish this off?" she asked.

"Usually what people say is, 'Would you like some more?'" I pointed out.

"I'm in my third trimester," she said.

I let her have it.

OCTOBER 23

On Thursdays I'm gone all day, don't get home until 9:00 or 9:30, and it's been interesting, if that's the word, to see each week how much harder these long days alone with Maeve must be for Maura. At this point, when I get home the house is a shambles, I can tell they've eaten out of cans—or maybe there were fish sticks—the dog's bladder is near bursting, and there's the sense that threats and bribes had been flung through the air very recently. Hey, putting things back in order while Maura and Maeve are asleep—washing the day's dishes, picking up stuffed dolls, walking the dog—is not really a bad way to unwind and ease my way back into the circus that is my home.

OCTOBER 26

We occasionally switch off babysitting with a couple down the street—one of them coming here or one of us going there. The job always starts after the kids are in bed, to make it easy on the babysitter. But last night, when it was our turn for freedom, I had my doubts about it being easy at all for Maura. She's rarely made it past 9:00 for the past three months. And it was hard to imagine her being able to wait so long for dinner.

"Oh," she said, having already solved the latter problem, "I'll eat dinner here with Maeve, too."

Once out in the restaurant, it didn't take long before we started feeling guilty about Lisa sitting in our quiet and cold house with no TV, not even a bag of potato chips, and so we hurried through all the topics that we should have been talking about regularly over the last few months but have barely had time for. How's the grieving going? How's our marriage? Have we handled this big crisis all right? What do you want to do for Christmas? What do we name this baby?

Maura pulled a couple of baby-name books from her purse and we perused them over dessert. The light was dim, and I squinted to see the books, sure at first that we ought to give the kid a common and sturdy name, something that sounds the way overalls look, to embrace his boyness, and then equally sure five minutes later that we should be artsy and funky, a little Frank Zappa-ish.

The grieving thing got Maura crying a little before our meals arrived, but she was actually crying over how good she felt about wearing her mother's engagement ring. They'd had to cut it off Gail's finger, but Maura had it resized and it looks just right on her, though it took me a few days to get used to it. Her own wedding ring is a thin jewel-less platinum band we got from an estate jeweler for a hundred bucks—just as much an aesthetic decision as a financial one. This ring of Gail's has been more of a comfort to Maura than anything else we brought back from Vermont. Several times I've walked into a room and come upon her staring at it with what seems to be tranquility.

"And how's your grieving going?" she asked politely.

I shrugged, unable to describe how heavily it weighs on me at moments, how sometimes it's impossible to conceive of Gail's absence. "I'm sad about it all at least part of each day," I admitted. "It's even worse—or more poignant, anyway—when I see it affecting you, or how Maeve's incorporated it into her worldview."

I told her about yesterday when Maeve and I were at the bookstore, standing in line. She was right next to me and said, "Daddy, I'm just the right height for you to rest your arm on my head." I told her that now that I knew that, she couldn't grow up.

"Oh, Daddy, everybody has to grow up," she said.

"But it's still kind of sad," I said.

"Daddy," she said, hugging my leg, "when I grow up, and even when I'm a teenager, I'll always stay with you, if you're still alive."

Maura smiled at the story. "Don't die," she said.

OCTOBER 28

Really, you don't get a lot of time in this life to dwell on one thing. Perry had the spotlight to himself for a week or two, but then he had to give it up for Gail. Now Gail is edging to the back of the stage so that the little kid can come forward. No one's leaving completely, of course. They all lurk back there by the curtain, and come out for an occasional and quick dance, but I'm finding that it's easier to have a series of distinct emotions rather than try to see the entire stage at once. I have no idea how someone who has, say, triplets plus a mother with Alzheimer's would have one manageable minute per day.

OCTOBER 30

Read yesterday that Paul McCartney is a new father, another guy in his sixties plunging in again. I'm thinking—maybe because right now it's 5:00 in the morning and I'm wide awake—that being really old when you have a kid has the big advantage that you don't need much sleep. All those old people shuffling around their houses in the middle of the night could get part-time jobs as graveyard-shift babysitters. Supplement the Social Security a little.

OCTOBER 31

Maura turns forty next week. My own fortieth seems so long ago that it's hard to remember whether I thought twice about it, because I certainly don't about my birthdays now. As my sister Kathy says, "After forty, who cares?" But I'm picking up signals that forty does carry some weight for Maura, and that it would be wise for me to know it. She hasn't come right out and said so to me, but she did to Jennifer, who was asking her on the phone yesterday for suggestions and whether presents had to be extra-special this year.

"She said yes," said Jennifer. "No socks. No turtlenecks."

"So we're in what . . . the diamond-earring range?" I asked, half joking.

"You might want to assume so," said Jen.

Also, Maura *did* tell me last night that she's been thinking lately about how her mom always got her something really nice for her birthday, and that she always looked forward to it. I'm sure it was a statement about missing her mother rather than about me having to pick up that slack. Still. Tomorrow I go shopping.

I'd wanted to give Maura a party—a real blowout with all of our friends—but after an initial temptation to accept, she's decided no.

"I've been the center of attention too much already," she said. What she's looking forward to is maternity leave — the eight weeks the college gives her, plus the other eight weeks she'll take as unpaid leave-of-absence, plus the regular summer off. Eight months total, to do nothing except take care of someone who needs it more than she does.

NOVEMBER 1

Halloween last night. The temperature was about sixty-five, and so for the first time in several years, the kids didn't have to wear parkas and mittens over their costumes. Instead, the moon was out, pumpkins glowed on every porch, and the street was filled with people. It was the perfect illustration of why we love this neighborhood. Ten years ago, I've heard, there were no kids at all in the neighborhood — just old folks in houses that were getting run down. Now there are twenty-nine kids on our three-block street alone. We'll make it an even thirty.

"You want to be a streetwalker or a dealer tonight?" I asked Maura when we were deciding who would stay home to give out candy and who would take Maeve on her rounds.

"Do I look like I'm in any shape to be a streetwalker?" she said.

NOVEMBER 2

Two months to go. Death is a little less in the air and the new life is beginning to exert its influence. Maeve and I were talking yesterday about the baby screaming once it's born, and I joked that it was probably screaming inside Maura's belly right now. And it does feel as if that noise is just under our auditory range, like the really low rumble that used to precede the beginnings of Elvis's concerts.

The kid is flinging himself from side to side and top to bottom in Maura's belly. I asked her if he ever throws her off-balance, and she said he didn't except sometimes when she's trying to get out of bed and he decides to go in the other direction.

"Give him another month so he has more weight to throw around," I said, but she pointed out that by then he won't have enough room to get a running start. Isn't it amazing how nature thinks of these things?

NOVEMBER 3

My mom spent last week in Illinois with Jennifer and Andy, holding the new baby while they mowed the lawn and balanced their checkbook. One night Jennifer was able to get nine hours of sleep, then all the next day floated around the house as if she were on drugs. At the end of the week, when Jen and Andy were thanking her profusely for her help, my mom told them through her sentimental tears, "It should've been your mother here."

My mom, the traveling nanny, will be here no later than January 5.

NOVEMBER 4

It's a weepy evening. Maura began crying not long after I got home, strung out over, she said, not having gotten anything of substance done during the day. Sometimes the day fritters away, and panic sets in, and having taken your daughter to ballet class doesn't quite compensate for other wasted hours. Then she held up her finger, the nail of which is brown from a fungus. "And I'm old," she wept, "and I have to buy this old person's medicine at the drugstore."

I eased her upstairs so she could grade some papers and feel worthwhile, and when she was gone, Maeve began crying in frustration over trying to write a note to her teacher and forgetting which letters made the *ch* sound. It took a while to convince her that she could just cross out her mistake and continue on. Then she cried twice more before dinner was finally ready and Maura came back downstairs, composed and even almost smiling.

Maura had a small glass of wine with dinner, which I've begun to heartily endorse, especially on days like this. We take heart from what our friend Bonnie told us about her first pregnancy. Her OB was a surly French guy, and she'd nervously asked him whether it would be okay if she drank an occasional glass of wine. "Of course," he said impatiently, "unless you zhink all French women are idiots."

NOVEMBER 5

Another checkup today. This time we met with the other doctor in the office, just in case he's the one on call when the time comes. He didn't give any indication of being a right-wing nutcase. (Nor, for that matter, has our own doctor.) But we do know his views on VBAC—a vaginal birth after caesarean—because he spent most of the appointment pleasantly telling us all of the things that could go wrong if Maura decides to have one. Last time she didn't dilate at all, even after thirty-six hours of labor, and so she'd had the C-section. The last I heard, she's leaning this time toward going natural, though that would mean going *really* natural. With a VBAC, the scar from the previous surgery can rupture, and one of the signs of that happening is pain at the scar site. To be able to feel the pain means no drugs, no epidural.

There are enough other risks, this doctor tells us, to warrant some heavy thinking. The fact, for instance, that the placenta could rupture and the baby could be without blood for the five minutes or more it takes them to get Maura to an OR and get the baby out.

Maura sat kind of impassively while the doctor talked, not giving away what she was thinking. We haven't had a chance to talk about it ourselves since then—maybe this weekend when we go out to a restaurant for her birthday, just the kind of romantic dinner conversation you're reduced to when you have about twenty quiet and awake minutes a week to cover every important aspect of your lives.

My preference is for whatever doesn't get either of them killed or made into a vegetable. The doctor was decidedly unhelpful on that. "The C-section is definitely the safest thing for the baby," he said. "On the other hand, if we knew everything was going to go okay, then natural birth is the safest thing for the mother. I'll support whichever you choose."

NOVEMBER 6

We've been parents of one kid for so long that it sometimes feels that having a second will elevate Maura and me to a rarefied, even saintly, status in the parenting world. The change looms huge in our lives, in our conceptions of ourselves as parents. Then I do something like go to a school board meeting, as I did the other night, and listen to the superintendent ask who has multiple kids who'll be affected by a new rezoning plan the board's considering. I was almost the only one whose hand didn't go up.

"If you're going to try for three or four kids," Maura's doctor said at her checkup yesterday," I'd recommend the VBAC this time, because repeat C-sections can begin to cause problems."

"We're trying for two," Maura told him flatly.

NOVEMBER 7

Maura has turned forty, and has handled it with great aplomb, dressing herself in elegant black and charging into the day with something that looked to me like fortitude. What else is there to do? She didn't say anything about feeling old or about the fungus under her fingernail. With a profile like a Klee line, she looked vibrantly young.

Maeve hounded her to open her presents first thing in the morning, even though the hour between everyone getting out of bed and then hustling Maeve to the bus stop already strains with tasks that take three times as long as they should — getting dressed, brushing teeth, peeing. Still, I put two on the table next to the bowls of cereal I poured for all of us — one present from Maeve and one from my parents. Maeve's was a colorful wool scarf, and my parents' was socks — complemented, luckily, by a generous gift certificate to Ann Taylor.

I wanted to save my gift for calmer and more sentimental circumstances, but Maeve kept insisting, "Daddy has to give you his present."

"He's going to save his for this evening," Maura said softly, trying to head off a screaming protest and, probably, talk herself into waiting through the entire day.

"Well, I'm not sure where I put it," I said, getting up and pretending to be confused. "Oh, here it is in the candy dish."

And it was just like the TV commercial after she wrested the little box away from Maeve so she could open it herself: tears in her eyes, quivering lip, her arms around my neck, her voice catching so that she could barely whisper, "I hope you didn't break the bank."

I shrugged off her worry, and she didn't say anything again about it, clearly not interested in hearing just how much diamond earrings of that size cost.

NOVEMBER 10

I'm depressed. I don't know why, except that it's Monday morning and Maeve doesn't have school because . . . well, I don't even know why.

It doesn't matter. I thought Maura wasn't going to be teaching today, and I lay in bed this morning planning how I'd spend my part of the day, then I realized that Maura *does* teach, and that she has to leave early because she's got a meeting, and that when she gets home I have to go to a meeting, and so the day's pretty much shot before it even begins. This is not the kind of generous dad I want to be, but there it is. Part of the blues comes from the fact that yesterday Maeve was gone all day—with a friend and her parents to a children's museum in another town—and I got a lot done, but it was all out in the yard—mowing, thinning a bed of day lilies—and I thought today I'd do the more sit-at-the-desk kind of things that I have to have done by tomorrow when I teach, but sometimes it's almost impossible to do those things with Maeve here. Maybe she'll be in one of her coloring moods, and we'll work quietly across from each other at the kitchen table for hours. I don't know what Plan B would be. Schlep her to a park or something while I dwell on what else I could be doing.

All right, that paragraph's out, and now I'll see if I can overcome it. Be in the here and now with Maeve.

NOVEMBER 11

I ran out of steam yesterday, and then shut down so completely that I couldn't even tell Maura why I wasn't talking to her—or not talking beyond one-word answers to her questions. "Fine" was about the extent of my conversation for thirty-six hours, and that in a surly tone. It was like not being able to breathe, only mental.

Not that it was her, but it *was* all that birthday last week, beginning with realizing that a nice wool dust mop (which, in fact, we need and Maura would appreciate because of her allergies) wouldn't cut it. There wasn't any time last week that I didn't feel pretty good about making Maura Queen for a Day and then re-electing her for seven or eight consecutive terms, but the energy was just draining out some hole without me even knowing it. Then in the middle of a long afternoon yesterday with Maeve, the shut-off came. There were late signs, such as me letting Maeve stay in her pajamas until 2:00 just to avoid the protest over her getting dressed. But I had no resources to help me change course—such as going out for a beer with a buddy and letting off all the steam to him. There wasn't even a beer in the house that I could gulp down by myself, and the gigantic hassle of getting Maeve to the store so I could buy some was simply beyond my comprehension. Maura got no warning and no explanation when she got home. Just "fine."

"You know what?" Maura said today when I was finally able to sputter out a reason for the cold shoulder. "By about last Wednesday or Thursday, I began to feel like I really didn't want anyone to take care of me. I was ready to do things myself."

Well, another example of our stiff upper lips, each of us enduring what must be done.

The only good thing to come out of it was that I agreed with Ann, our friend from school, that she should throw me a birthday party next month. Actually, she originally proposed it as a shower for Maura, but when I told her it would be my birthday and that I could really use a little focus on me, we cut Maura out of the picture. Or at least I did. To hear Ann describe the department's last baby shower, about four years ago, it sounds as if Maura and I could go to this party and each easily see it as our own little evening of adoration. The last one wasn't some women-only thing. Everyone was invited. "We all drank way too much," Ann said. "Most of us really didn't know anyone before that who'd, like, had kids, and so people were bringing presents like lamps. It was great."

NOVEMBER 12

Most of the time now when we call Jennifer and Andy out in Illinois, there are screaming kids in the background and Jennifer's saying, curtly and with the smallest hint of panic in her voice, "This is not a good time to talk."

This is definitely a bad sign of things to come.

NOVEMBER 13

Two days ago I was painting the fence in the warm midday sun, and this morning at the bus stop we were all bundled in snowboots and parkas. It snowed most of yesterday and last night, and it's cold cold cold out, and the wind's blowing forty miles an hour. My mom theorized on the phone that the boy, once he gets a whiff of the Syracuse winter, will grow up and move to Hawaii, which will be good for us because we'll have a warm place to visit. "Nah," I said, "he'll never leave. We'll have to keep telling him, 'Go away!'" But I'm just hoping that a winter birth will make him tough—that he won't, like all those northerners who move south, be on a wimpy lifelong search to recapture the warmth of the womb.

NOVEMBER 14

Maybe I need to read some child psych books about girls. At some moments, I begin to think that Maura's OB might have been right—that you have to talk to girls like adults, that you never really know what they're thinking, and that it's all just a whole lot of trouble. I don't think this way often, but every once in a while, Maeve goes into some territory that I'm simply not allowed into, like a scary parallel world. Monday afternoon, for instance. She'd had a wonderful morning at school, had gotten off the bus happy and run into my arms, had sloughed off her jacket and left it charmingly on the living room floor, then retrieved it and tossed it on her bed when I reminded her that it was supposed to be hung on the hook in her room. She plopped herself down at the kitchen table and began drawing with her markers. I love those domestic moments—me making her some lunch, the two of us chatting happily, the wonderful afternoon stretching out before us. I figured we'd take a walk later, bake cookies, laugh, feel mutually satisfied and shining with father-daughter love when Maura got home, envious over the perfect world into which she trudges. I was cutting Maeve's grilled cheese into triangles when she let out a little cry of frustration. She'd been drawing a connect-the-dots heart, and on the dot where she meant to put a 13, she'd accidentally begun to draw a 12. I walked over and tried to show her how she could simply make the 2 into a 3 with a tail, but that only upset her more. I suggested—gently, with my best loving voice—that it was only a tiny mistake, not even a mistake really but an opportunity for creativity.

"What if you put another dot between those and make that 12, then the other one can be 13?"

She wailed as if I'd suggested she rip it all up and start again. "If I do that, then the connect the dots won't be like I want it."

"Well, you can put the dot exactly in the middle, so the line will be just the same as it would've been before."

"But, Daddy, then the dot will make a bump in the line, and it won't look like I want it to."

I put our lunches on the table and began eating, hoping her own food would distract her. When it didn't, I tried to suggest other solutions, until the only conclusion was that there were no solutions. I decided to wait it out.

"I'm going to sit here without talking, because whenever I say something, that seems to make you madder," I said.

"Daddy, when you talk it does make me mad," she wailed, "but I also get mad when you don't talk."

She was backing both of us into a corner, and we were juking around each other.

Last year she occasionally went into phases like this, fascinated by worst-case scenarios, and we'd have conversations like this one:

"Maeve, you've got to eat up and brush your teeth because we have to leave for school in ten minutes. Let's hurry up."

"But what if I was sick and I couldn't go to school?" she'd ask.

"Then someone would have to stay home with you. But you're not sick, so let's get a move on."

"But what if you had to go to school and Mommy had to go to school and I was sick?"

"Then one of us would stay home with you."

"But what if you had to go to school?"

"Then Grandma Gail would come and stay with you."

"But what if Grandma Gail was sick and couldn't come?"

"Then Grandma Bonnie would come and stay with you."

"But what if everybody was sick and couldn't come?"

"Then Aunt Theresa or someone else would come and stay with you."

"But what if *everybody* was sick?"

"Then I guess you'd have to stay by yourself."

"But kids don't stay by themselves."

"Then I'd stay home with you. I'd quit my job and stay home."

I could never tell what answer she ultimately wanted, how far I had to go into absurdity before she'd be satisfied. Usually, it ended with Maura and me devoting ourselves completely and absolutely to her care. Was this normal? Was there some hidden message here that we weren't already doing everything we needed for her?

The conversation today was along those lines but with the tension ratcheted up to explosive levels.

"Maeve, what can I *do* for you that will make you feel better?" I finally asked.

That question didn't even seem right—the wrong tone. *Patience*, I said silently, and I remembered a moment when Maeve was two and accomplished exactly what I was trying to accomplish now. She had her eleven-month-old friend Clementine over. Clemmie was lonely for her mom, and I could do nothing to get her to stop crying. Maeve kept saying, "Let's bring her some orange juice" or "Does Clemmie want to go outside?" She was concerned but never rattled. She gave Clemmie hugs, kept trying to get her to laugh. Brought her books. And finally, after nearly two hours, Maeve began playing catch with her, sitting in the kitchen rolling the ball back and forth, and the two girls couldn't stop laughing. Cracking up. When Clemmie's mom came to get her, she didn't want to leave. *Live up to that standard*, I told myself.

"Daddy, I'm crying because there's *nothing* you can do for me."

"Can I give you a hug? Would that help?"

She walked around the table toward me, then began hitting me. She took some good swings, and let out sharp and frustrating screams at the same time, like a small martial artist. I couldn't let her simply hit me, and so I tried to stop that without making things worse.

"Now, you can't hit someone when you're mad," I tried to explain, as matter-of-factly as I could.

She stared at me and screamed in short bursts. When I got up to put my lunch dishes in the sink, she went hysterical because she thought I was leaving. Instead, I went back to the digesting chair and coaxed her over, slowly got her to get on my lap so I could hug her. She was still crying, but ever so slowly she began to relax, and she put her head down on my shoulder when I encouraged her to. I rubbed her back, cooing that everything was all right. We stayed like that for twenty minutes, letting the tension ease. I felt so bad for her.

And then it was gone. The rest of the afternoon passed as if nothing had ever happened. I have no idea.

Looking back on it now, all I can think is that I handled it the best I could, that I'd been somewhat tested and proven my adequacy, though maybe not my excellence. But I'm filled with wariness, remembering what a friend of mine who has two college-age daughters told me recently: "Wait till the hormones kick in. It's going to turn your gray hair brown."

NOVEMBER 15

I'm now a great-uncle. Ryan and Karen have had their baby, a little girl they've named Bailey. They were at the hospital for hours without Karen dilating, and when the doctors finally decided to induce her, Ryan excused himself and said he had to go home and get the stroller. "You're not going to need the stroller for a while yet," my mom told him gently.

It sounds like it was Grand Central Station in the birth suite — about fifteen people, including four kids. Karen apparently didn't care, just screamed and moaned as if no one were there. I have to admit that I'm attracted to the idea of making the birth be such a party. Less fun things like hangings and whippings have had their days as public events, while birthing women have usually had to hide away in tents and bulrushes and Authorized-Persons-Only operating rooms, after which someone carries out a kid that's as clean as a plastic doll. Maybe it's because Karen's only twenty and dreamy that she could turn the event into a real birthday party. Or maybe she simply feels so close to her family, and is relying so much on them to help her make it through motherhood, that she wants them there for everything. It's hard to argue with that wisdom.

I know I won't be elbowing any other spectators out of my way when it's Maura's turn. When I told her about the crowd she said, "Well, that's an interesting personal choice."

NOVEMBER 17

Our friends Bonnie and Mike, the Foreign Service cowboys, finish their Bulgarian tour next summer and have found out where they go next. One possibility was Paris, another was Frankfurt, and of course we'd been angling for first crack at their guest quarters. Amazingly, they didn't even *ask* for those places. Their top choice, which — surprise! — they got, was Bangladesh. Something like seventy percent of the country floods each year. "Our house will be on high ground," Bonnie assured us in an email. Well, I'm impressed by what their kids will know of the world by the time they're ten, but I have to say that I don't see us packing up Maeve and a baby for a visit to Dhaka in the next three years.

We had some decent snows yesterday and today—two inches followed by four inches—which makes Bangladesh feel all that much further away.

NOVEMBER 19

Waking up in the morning is a comic act this week. I've got some disgusting cyst under my arm that feels—when the painkillers wear off—like what I've read a gunshot wound feels like, and it takes me six or eight tries to get out of bed: pushing and pulling with my good arm and my weak stomach muscles while holding my bad arm absolutely still. Maura takes deep breaths and starts slowly like a shot-putter before she can overcome her own inertia. If there were a baby in a crib on the other side of the room needing us, he'd have to scream for a couple minutes before help arrived.

The dog, of course, flops around so much in trying to stand up that he usually cracks his hard head against the wood floor. When he's finally up on all four feet, he looks dazed and his fur goes in all directions, but then he seems fine.

Maeve's the only one capable of hopping out of bed, but she doesn't because, as she whined this morning, "I'm still tired."

NOVEMBER 22

We're beginning to feel the enlargement of vision that comes with having a second kid. I'm not sure this vision is reliable, or healthy, and it feels like one of those cultural pressures that weigh on you without your wanting it or consciously asking for it, like the pressure to dress your son in blue or not to wear earth shoes anymore even if you've saved them in a box for the last thirty years.

The vision has to do with space. Maura and I have been walking around the house, trying to imagine what the living arrangements will be like in six months, in six years, in ten years. Maeve's got a tiny room that she seems to inhabit perfectly right now, but if she's still in there when she's seven or eight or ten, she'll probably have some dented tin cup that she'll bang against the wall while she yells, "Attica! Attica!" Her sense of humor is already gaining a sarcastic edge.

And the fact that this next kid will be a boy doesn't make it easy to imagine that a small house will be enough. There's a reason besides alliteration, isn't there, that they always refer to baby boys as "bouncing"? Also, none of the boys in my family is small. My brother Pat is six-foot-four and weighs 250. What if we get one of those?

So we're thinking about an addition — just the kind of thing that *New Yorker* article a few months ago said contributed to married couples with children going bankrupt. We wouldn't even be thinking about it, alas, if Gail hadn't died, because I don't see how we could swing it. We'd have to make do with what we've got — which is probably a healthy way to live. But now we've got a little pile of cash from Gail's estate — the very money she had saved for her retirement and never got to use. We both have very mixed feelings about spending it on ourselves. The only way we can rationalize it is that we had talked to Gail about doing this very thing. We'd been encouraging her to sell the house in Vermont, use part of the profit to build her own addition on to our house, and live there. She wanted a smaller place, we wanted her close, and she was seriously considering the idea. It would've been cheaper for her than buying a condo — though not as warm as moving to Florida, which she claimed (unconvincingly, I thought) she wanted to do.

Besides, now that Vermont is no longer the gathering place for Maura's side of the family, we'd like to make our home into that place — people hanging out here for Christmas, for a couple weeks each summer, for any other time they want to come. It would be nice if they didn't have to sleep foot-to-foot like Charlie Bucket's family.

So this afternoon I'm going to call an architect, see what the process might be like. It makes me nostalgic for the days before kids, when the rule of thumb was: Don't own anything more than will fit in your car.

NOVEMBER 23

People are telling Maura she's dropped. This is only part of the attention she gets from everyone, including the garbageman. He was riding on the back of the truck while Maura was out for a walk this morning, and he looked her up and down for a block and then yelled, "That baby's going to be a boy, isn't it?" Lucky guess.

A premature baby would not be good, not only because of the health issues, but because if the baby comes before, say, January 5, it'll cut into the maternity leave that Maura gets for the spring semester. Classes start on January 9, and if the baby's on time, Maura gets the maximum paid leave possible.

I heard on the radio yesterday that of the 113 babies typically born each week in this county, thirteen of them are premature, and one of them dies. Stats like this only add to the stress. Maura asked her doctor about it, and he had his typical calming words. Women tend to drop earlier the second time, because the muscles are all stretched out. Don't sweat it. I'm sure that eased Maura's mind as much as did the doctor's assurance that her newly arrived varicose veins will probably go away after the birth.

NOVEMBER 24

Maeve came in to get me last night, at about 12:30, while I was in the middle of a dream about, I think, California. She had her usual line, that she was scared of the dark, and I couldn't generate any enthusiasm for taking her back to her bedroom and lying in bed with her. After a minute or two, though, with her standing over me the way I stand over her in the morning, I dragged myself up. I held her hand and we inched around the dog, who takes up the entire floor between the foot of the bed and the closet. I wasn't very pleasant company for her, I'm sure, but I stayed under her covers until she fell back asleep, then dragged myself up again for the reverse trip. At moments like those I always remember the WW I soldier I read about as a kid, in one of those "strange but true" books: a bullet had zinged past his temple, scraping it just enough to hit the sleep controls in his brain, and he lost all need to sleep. He apparently wasn't a parent, and so he adopted a routine of spending the nights in different bars, chatting away, and only needed to sit in his recliner every once in a while to rest his eyes. The book said he ultimately got bored with his life, because nobody else could keep up with him. It was a completely whacko book, of course, though I remember trying to will myself into believing the story, simply because I wanted to feel jealous of the guy. And if the story had one iota of truth to it, my jealousy would now be ratcheted up considerably.

NOVEMBER 25

The semester is winding down, which means that Maura and I are on the old path of coming back together, seeing each other a bit more, actually having time to talk and hang out. That's all fine, though it's not so easy getting close to Maura physically, because her belly is so big. I'm always dancing around her, trying to find an opening, like a wrestler. She naturally turns toward me, and the kid sits right between us.

NOVEMBER 26

It looks as if we'll spend this Thanksgiving week focused on caring for a sick kid. Maeve woke up at 2:00 last night with a fever and headache so bad that she was sitting in bed and screaming, holding her arms straight and raising and lowering them as if she were doing the wave. It took two minutes before I could get her to calm down enough to confirm that her head was the cause of the screaming, rather than some nightmare or cramp in her foot. Her skin was as hot as if she'd spent two hours in a Jacuzzi. When she could finally talk, I asked her if she'd been dizzy, and she said, through shallow breaths, "Daddy, it felt like I was flying."

Maeve is sick so rarely that in between the episodes I forget what's it's like. So it's creepy to see her helpless, and this time I immediately remembered that woman I'd taken to the hospital in the ambulance months ago, and I thought: *meningitis*. I had Maeve touch her chin to her chest. She could. So I patted her down with a cool cloth, got her to take some grape-flavored Tylenol, and let her fall back asleep. When she woke up screaming an hour and a half later, I did it all again, except for the medicine.

NOVEMBER 27

Maura was sitting on the stairs a little while ago, in her warm boots, with a scarf around her neck, looking as if she might be getting ready to go for a walk in the new snow. Or she could've been simply catching her breath.

"What are you doing?" I asked.

"Meditating upon a life misspent," she said.

"It's Thanksgiving," I pointed out. "You're supposed to be giving thanks."

"Okay. Thank you, God, for taking my mother at a time when I could least afford it. Thank you for my daughter's sickness." She looked out the window and figured she'd better tone it down. "Thank you for the nice day."

I can't keep up with her when she decides to get sarcastic.

NOVEMBER 28

I'm baking a chocolate-cream pie. Maura's sister Sheila, who is visiting for the week, is sitting on the sofa writing in her notebook. Maeve is listless in bed, listening to Rosemary Clooney sing Christmas carols. Maura is out for a walk. The dog is sleeping in the hostas out front. It promises to be a quiet day.

It's very cold outside, but Maeve's temperature peaked at 105 this afternoon, and she was absolutely wilted. I got some medicine into her, then carried her upstairs for a lukewarm sponge bath. She moaned and writhed through both of them, but within an hour her fever came down two degrees, and within another hour it was actually down to 98.6. She was bouncing around the house and laughing, teasing Sheila. It's amazing how much a fever saps you, but there are moments when, if we hadn't had the thermometer to give us some real numbers, I don't think I'd have been as forebearing with much of Maeve's seeming discomfort. For instance, at one of her worst moments, I carried her out to the kitchen to try to get her to eat a little something, and I'd just poured her some orange juice. I was holding her on my hip near the sink and she was sobbing as if someone were pulling her toenails out, and then she stopped instantly and said in a perfectly normal voice, "The refrigerator door is not closed all the way, Daddy." "Oh, thank you for letting me know," I said. "You're welcome," she said pleasantly. Then she resumed the same sobbing as before. I get a little suspicious.

NOVEMBER 29

It's the next day, and once again the night was punctuated by Maeve waking up with piercing screams that jolted me out of bed without any thought of the lingering pain from that underarm cyst. We went through the routine—the calming, the Tylenol, the bringing her into bed to sleep with me while Maura trudged off alone to Maeve's bed like the Jeff Goldblum character in *The Big Chill*—and this morning Maeve felt good enough to be kicking me in bed and poking me in the cheek. I'd slept fitfully, waking up every now and then to hear Maura coughing or running a hot shower to clear her lungs. She dragged herself out of bed about 8:30 and trudged grimly to the bathroom. When she passed by me, she looked both angry and completely put out. I really tried to empathize when she complained that she hadn't gotten to sleep until 6:30, but I was tired too, and the compassion just wasn't springing from my heart like it should've been.

My empathy did spike a bit in the afternoon, when my brother Steve called from Los Angeles to say that all three of his daughters were sick at once—and not with mere runny noses but with ugly, messy, give-them-up-for-adoption things like infections and diarrhea. The girls are five, three, and ten months. I didn't even want to think about it. I just rang it up as another Southern California disaster that I could avoid if I never move there—like a wildfire, an earthquake, or a half-million dollar two-bedroom house.

NOVEMBER 30

"It's not twice as much work, but it *is* three times as much laundry." So said our friend Cindy, who has a seven-year-old boy and a five-year-old girl. I'm not sure I believe her about the work, but I can already hear the constant chug of the washing machine.

Someone else told me once that having two kids *is* twice as much work, but it's also four times as much fun—an apparently good trade-off in that person's book.

This idea of logarithmic multiplicity is what's leading us, I think, to consider adding three or four more rooms to the house when we actually only need one more. Two kids are going to occupy four or five times as much space, in the way that two wolves do because they have to roam their own territories.

What else is going to quadruple rather than double? The noise in the house? Our food bill? Probably this last one, since Maeve eats like a pet garter snake, the equivalent of a worm a week.

What I hope goes *down* is the level of fear and protectiveness that Maura and I have as parents. I have only the tiniest bit of optimism for this, and only because of a line I read years ago in Patricia Hampl's memoir *A Romantic Education*, in which she is describing her grandmother, who, when she was babysitting the young Hampl, would let her be gone for hours without wondering or seemingly caring where she was. "She had the casualness of someone who'd had ten kids," Hampl wrote.

My friend Karl, who is famous in our circles for blunt remarks that he *thinks* people want to hear, once said that one of the best reasons for having a second kid is in case the first one dies. Now, in a good part of the world this is no doubt true, but this was not the kind of reasoning I wanted to weave into our own deliberations. In those rare moments when I'm able to imagine the absolute horror of Maeve dying young, there is nothing—not even my own son—who could be a substitute. Or anything *like* a substitute. All I can imagine—in my poor, optimistic mind that has never been traumatized by the loss of something so close (not a cat, for sure, and not, I'm afraid, a mother-in-law)—is that I would live the rest of my life with a gigantic and unfillable hole, and that I would spend hours each day poring over the hundreds of pictures I've already taken of Maeve, more hours scrutinizing every drawing of hers we've saved, more hours simply crying, more hours writing her painful letters that I would not know what to do with once they were done. I fear it would ruin me as a father.

Still. There is, I admit, just the tiniest bit of insurance-policy thinking in my subconscious. It's risky to go through life with a small family, in the same way it's risky to go through it skinny. You want some reserves to fall back on, if only to make you feel slightly better about yourself after you've spent time thinking like an actuary rather than like a parent.

A nice snow—four or five inches—to end the month. I hadn't expected this much snow this early in the season, and I've got to get on the ball with a project I should already be far along on—the building of an ice rink in the backyard. I'd intended to put the thing together over Thanksgiving weekend—it involves driving some wooden stakes into the ground and attaching two-by-twelves to form a big rectangle, then stapling in a huge plastic sheet to hold the water—but I haven't even bought the two-by-twelves yet. Today, I'm off to the lumber store.

DECEMBER 1

Maura's had a chest cold for about ten days, so at her checkup this morning her doc gave her a script for some drugs.

He also pointed out, though we already knew, that she's now at thirty-five weeks. "One more week and you'll be considered full-term," he said, telling us something we hadn't thought about.

That news was scary enough, but then he threw out the statistic again about VBAC—the one-percent chance of the old incision rupturing—as a way to find out what Maura's thinking these days about how to get this baby out. But he toned down the dire predictions from what his partner had laid on us, emphasizing that the chance of the uterus bursting open for Maura is about the same as for a woman having her fourth or fifth kid vaginally.

"I'm thinking VBAC," Maura said.

"So we'll do it in the hospital, and we'll watch closely," the doctor said, in his best soothing voice.

"Just in case the baby's as big as Maeve was?" Maura asked.

"Hey, I've seen a mother have a C-section with a small baby, then have a VBAC with a nine-pounder and have the kid slip right out," he said. "It drives you nuts. It's not size that's important, but position. If the head's down where it should be in the pelvic bone, things tend to go pretty well. But if it's a little to the side, there's not much you can do. Last night I did a section, and the baby was only six and a half pounds."

I wondered aloud whether this bad positioning was the reason women used to die so frequently during childbirth.

"You mean in the 'olden days'?" the doctor said, smiling. "That was only 1940, when antibiotics began to be used. Before that, mothers who had a C-section would often die of sepsis. You know—and people don't appreciate this—modern medicine is only sixty years old. Back in our grandmother's time, life was hard. If you got whooping cough, you died. If you got the flu, you probably died. If you had a C-section, chances were you died."

"Remember that movie *Restoration*," Maura said, "where Robert Downey Jr. is a seventeenth-century doctor who does a C-section on his wife, and beforehand, he says goodbye?"

"That was it," the doctor chimed in, excited about the tragedies of medical history. "Back then they also did what was called a destructive procedure. You go up in there and cut up the fetus and take it out part by part, to save the uterus. It was a hard, hard life."

I saw an opening. "As long as we're on worst-case scenarios," I said, "let me ask you a philosophical question. Or a pragmatic one. Maybe I shouldn't ask it with Maura sitting here."

She sighed and waved me on, knowing immediately what I had in mind.

"Go ahead," said the doctor.

"At this point in a pregnancy, or really at any point, if there's trouble of some serious kind, how do you decide which patient gets priority—the mother or the baby?"

"You mean who do you save?"

"Well, okay."

"We don't even ask that question these days. If something happens that endangers the baby, we get it out. We save them both. Look, I did my training at an abortion hospital. Not that I *did* them, but they were all around. And even there, I never saw—and the old-timers had never seen—a case where you had to sacrifice the mother to save a viable baby, or vice versa. It just doesn't happen. So all this stuff about late-term abortions—partial-birth abortions, I guess they call them—is crap. Purely a moneymaker. It's a political question, not a medical one."

Then he changed the subject.

"So," he said to Maura, "what can you do to bring on contractions? Intercourse. Seminal fluid helps to relax the cervix." He put his hand on my shoulder and smiled at Maura. "I'm sure you've got a brave man here, someone not afraid he's going to hurt the baby."

I shrugged modestly. "Wherever I'm needed," I said. At this point the last time around, Maura's OB had told me, "If there's nothing on TV, you can play with her nipples."

"So, we call you when . . . ?" Maura asked.

"When your water breaks. When there's bleeding. When you've got regular contractions—at least ten minutes apart for an hour. Or if you have questions. If you're not sure whether to call or not, call."

He sent us off. "Keep thinking about those big philosophical questions," he told me.

DECEMBER 2

It's the last week of classes for this semester. All the real work is done, and now it's just a matter of tying up loose ends — collecting final papers, figuring grades. Likewise, there seems little left to do with the pregnancy. We've survived the scares, the tensions, the miscarriages, the exhaustions — and now it feels out of our hands.

Even with this feeling that we have nothing left to do but wait, we haven't wrapped everything up. We've left loose ends, and few things about this pregnancy are certain, even now. What about that funny little thing in the kid's heart? It was still there the last time we looked. We've really just written it off like a birthmark, trusting that it's either gone away or will never cause any problems. Who knows? And what about an unlimited number of other possible birth defects? Sure, all the limbs and digits show up on the ultrasound, and they look like they're the right sizes, but what about things no one can see until the kid comes out? When I came out, lo and behold, my right eye had this cataract smack dab on the pupil. (No one seemed to know what to do with it, and so I'm blind in that eye today.) What about the kid's blood? His genetic makeup? His alveoli, or capillaries, or hair follicles, or dura mater, or other minuscule body parts that could be horribly disfigured and broken? Getting an ultrasound is really just like getting your car inspected, isn't it? They make sure the horn honks, the brake lights work, and the turn signals blink, but you could drive away with your new sticker shining in the window and have the transmission seize up on you.

DECEMBER 3

The last time we got to this point, we were finishing our Lamaze class, panicking over the impossibility of remembering the details of infant CPR. We'd finish the lesson and then on the way home ask each other, "So, do you hold the kid upside down or right-side-up?" A few weeks ago Maura wondered whether we should go through a refresher course. "Nah," I said, partly because I've done the EMT training and partly because it would be embarrassing to take the class now. Last time we were older than any other couple in the room by a decade. This time would only be much worse.

DECEMBER 4

Maura mentioned last night that the baby is no longer a part of her, but something separate that she happens to be hauling around in her belly, something she occasionally feels like putting down on the table and walking away from.

DECEMBER 5

I saw in the paper yesterday that there are only twenty-one shopping days left before Christmas, and I realized that the rest of the country is on a different countdown than we are. There's only one way to be able to live on both of these timelines, and that's to remove one from my head as soon as possible. Everyone's getting books this year. That's the theme. I'm going to make one trip down the street to our friend Nancy's children's bookstore and buy whatever she's got in stock, then I'll go once to a charming little independent bookstore out in Cazenovia and knock off all the adults on our list. After that, Christmas will arrive and pass like a small wave in a big ocean.

Things are getting interesting in bed these days. I reach over to see if Maura's there, if she's come back to bed after one of her coughing fits, and all I feel are pillows. She has one between her knees, one under her belly, a couple under her head. She's afloat on them like a goose on straw. If the baby came out now, it would land softly and comfortably, and would go right to sleep.

DECEMBER 6

Today I turn forty-five. In my mind has been a joke David Letterman cracked last month about becoming a father for the first time at fifty-six. "By the time he's old enough to steal cars," he said, "I'll be dead."

I'm currently feeling up to the task physically, anyway, and that's something. But it's impossible not to do the same kinds of calculations that Letterman did, and try to imagine if I'll have anything left by the time the kid wants to play catch. It's a hard picture to bring up.

Letterman's joke also got me thinking about how, as an older parent, pretty much the only thing you can do, if you want to approach this job with any semblance of sanity, is to keep your own abilities and timeline in perspective. God willing, you can give the kid a lot for a while — twenty years, I'd hope — and then it's out of your hands. You either voluntarily or involuntarily remove yourself from the picture.

I kind of like this . . . not a casualness, really, but an acceptance. A reconciliation with what's likely to happen. It's not that I now assume I'll be dead at sixty-five (a life-expectancy quiz I took recently has me cooking until ninety-eight) or that if I'm gone before that my kids would live on as comfortably and happily without me as would my cat. It's more that what happens, happens. Maura and I finally got around to making wills last spring, before we went to Ireland, and so we know that Jennifer and Andy get the kids if it comes to that. (We'll take theirs if they make an early exit.) There are other pragmatic things we can do, of course. We ought to get more life insurance. I ought to write down everything I'd ever want Maeve and her brother to know, in case I can't tell them in person. Who knows the extent to which either of these things will happen?

If I'd had kids in my twenties, I know that my sense of responsibility toward them would've been much more intense — a panicked kind of accountability, a fear that I'd have had to oversee *every*thing, and that it all would reflect back on me. And that I'd have to do it for, say, sixty years.

My entire conception of responsibility has changed over the years, and it probably shows up most right now in my teaching. I used to assume that I was more of my students' partner in their successes or failures. I did whatever I could — meeting extensively with them outside of class, giving extra comments on papers, allowing more time on assignments — to see that they learned the material, even if I knew that I was doing more work than they were. I'm *much* less patient now. Who's got time to hold their hands? Or the energy?

I suspect my switch from Mr. Rogers to drill sergeant came sometime after Maeve arrived, when my students were no longer the youngest people I saw on a regular basis. Who knows whether this change of attitude has made me a better teacher or a worse one—though I sometimes think that my impatience is telling me either that I ought to get a job in which I deal with more mature people, if there *is* such a job, or that I ought to work alone in a quiet room, in loneliness and poverty.

Inevitably, I'll make the same transition for Maeve as I have for my students, once she's no longer the youngest person in my world. I feel a little bad about laying this new heaviness on her, though not bad enough that Maura and I haven't already used it as tools in our manipulations. "You know," we've threatened her, "when your little brother comes along, I'm not going to have time to help you put on your socks every morning, so you might as well learn how to do it yourself now." She doesn't buy it.

One of the hardest things about having a new baby will be remembering that Maeve is still only five years old.

DECEMBER 7

All this birthday weekend I kept expecting Gail to call. It snowed six or eight inches.

No big birthday party.

DECEMBER 8

Maeve got engaged today. Her friend Curtis, who is in first grade, gave her a ring on the bus. Maeve showed it to me when I got home. "It's the most beautiful thing I ever could have wished for," she said wistfully, several times. It's in a little silver ring box, and Maeve flips it open to reveal what looks like a real ring.

Maura and I told her how happy we were for her. What can you do but play along? Curtis's mom, Lynniece, said that she tried to explain to Curtis that people grow up and change and don't always end up with the people they think they're going to. "Maybe," said Curtis earnestly, "but I really want to try to make this work."

This has all made me realize that perhaps this is a good time for me to have another kid. At bedtime tonight I told Maeve to dream only about me—a joke we've had running between us for a few months. "I'm going to dream about my wedding to Curtis," she said.

DECEMBER 9

I've spent much of the last two days in the backyard, trying to assemble the ice rink. I had my first rink last year, but it was an amateurish affair, with snowbanks along the perimeter rather than boards. Since there was no plastic to hold in the water, I had to build the ice up slowly—like a parfait, with micro-thin layers on the bottom and gradually thicker layers over the course of two or three days—on snow I'd packed down by jumping on a piece of plywood. It was a cold mess. The yellow plastic sprayer wouldn't screw tightly enough onto the hose, and water ran down my sleeve. The temperature during those days rarely cracked zero, and a stiff breeze kicked the spray back at me so that ice built up on my chest and legs as if I were the bow of an Arctic ship. Still, after it was all done, I got to skate on a backyard rink for the first time since I was a kid, and it hooked me. And Maeve, too, who learned to skate out there on that bumpy ice. I resolved I'd upgrade this year—smoother ice, more surface area. Hence, the boards.

But, damn, the snow doesn't make it easy. I rush out to pound some more stakes and screw more boards to them whenever it's not snowing, but pretty soon the flakes are coming down thick and fast. The drill bit starts getting stuck in the wood because the drill gets wet and loses its grip. I stomp inside to get the pliers, curse first under my breath and then loudly enough for the neighbors to hear, if anyone's listening. The summer before last I put together a swingset: four days of unrelenting profanity. It's ten times worse in the snow. Boards slip over each other, the snow melts on my glasses and forces me to tilt my head and look sideways at things, and my pants are wet from the knees down. But, you know, it's addictive. And there's no stopping now, because I've been boasting about the rink at the bus stop in the morning. Kids all over the neighborhood are asking when they'll be able to go skating at Maeve's house. I plow on.

DECEMBER 10

All of this snow—we're up to about fifty inches already, and it's still officially fall—has gotten me thinking in a different way about the wisdom of having a baby in the middle of a Syracuse winter. Months ago, I'd imagined us nesting comfortably, huddled inside and occasionally peering out the window to see how far the snow had built up and how long the icicles were on the eaves. I'd imagined an occasional stroll to the store to get some essential supplies, like marshmallows and brownie mix, plus an occasional and energizing trudge to the woodpile. Basically, we'd all exist for the first few months inside the amniotic sac of our house, the heat turned up and some Mozart playing quietly on the stereo. I'd have to leave now and then to go teach my classes, but I'd glide through those without any real disruption of our main routine. And when spring arrived, we'd emerge from the house along with the buds on the trees, and we'd enter without a ripple into the comfortable and easy northern summer.

Now I'm thinking of the complications. What if there's a blizzard on the day Maura goes into labor? (A likely scenario at this point.) And there's the dog, which of course we didn't plan on having but who needs to go out four or five times a day, so that the seal to our little sac is constantly broken, a cold breeze whooshing through the house and little clumps of snow melting throughout the kitchen and all along the path through the dining room to the coat closet by the front stairs. (I can't take off my boots *every* time I come in, because I usually need to go out again soon after.) Someone has to shovel the driveway and the sidewalk. And pretty soon the ice rink. Our lives are not as hard as that of the woman from whom we bought a Christmas tree the other day. She raises not only trees but also alpacas and some other unspecified critters, and the roof on her barn collapsed under the snow and so she has to make other arrangements for the animals before they freeze to death. Her driveway is half a mile long and she plows it herself. She seems to work several different jobs. Buying a tree from her not only put us in the Christmas spirit but also put our lives into a necessary perspective.

This week's *New Yorker* has a wonderful little essay by Louise Erdrich about having babies in the winter in Minnesota. She's found, now that her oldest daughters are teenagers, that her timing means horrible things like them learning to drive in the winter. "Because the oldest two both took the driver's test the days after their sixteenth birthday," she writes, "much of the practice driving—with learner's permits, and me riding as the requisite adult passenger—took place on those slush-ridden, black-iced, snowbound, or low-visibility Minnesota mornings as we made our way harrowingly to school." So much of the difficulty with kids seems to involve cars—as it does, in fact, with adults.

We're getting an infant car seat from our friends Tim and Lynniece down the street, if Emily grows out of it in the next couple of weeks. She's almost there, and so every time we see her we silently urge her, like a couple of strength coaches, to pack on the pounds and the inches.

DECEMBER 13

The frame of the rink has been finished for a week—taking up the front half of the backyard—a fifty-by-thirty-foot monstrosity. A couple people have spotted it from the street and said, "What *is* that?" It doesn't look like something that will increase anyone's property value. And everyone seems relieved when I explain that it's not permanent, that I'll take it all down in the spring, then put it back together next winter, and so on until the wood rots, I get sick of the job, or global warming makes upstate New York winters as warm as North Carolina's are now. Anyway, late yesterday afternoon I finally got a chance to spread the plastic over it, though I first had to shovel eight or ten inches out of the interior so I could get the plastic flush with the ground. It's the first time I've ever shoveled the grass.

DECEMBER 17

Today I filled the rink. And discovered some bad things along the way. Such as: the northwest corner is *way* lower than the southeast corner. I mean about sixteen inches. I knew this when I built the frame, because I had to add an extra two-by-twelve and then another two-by-four to the northwest corner to keep the top of the frame level all the way around and still have boards clear to the ground (essential for keeping water in and giving support to the plastic). But I didn't really consider it a big deal until I slung the garden hose over the boards and turned on the water. I let it run for *hours*. The low end filled slowly, and every time I'd check on the progress, three-quarters of the rink would still be above water. It was as if it were leaking out the low end. And then finally the water began to creep over more of the plastic, inching up the high parts. It took most of the day—and, I calculated, about ten thousand gallons—but by evening there was water throughout. It was only an inch deep in the southeast corner—plenty to skate on once it freezes — but it was seventeen inches deep in the other end. I can't imagine it *ever* freezing. Worse, the weight of all that water is pushing out on the frame where I've got two long boards butted together. I screwed in a couple extra metal brackets and pounded two more wooden stakes into the ground for support. I have no idea if it'll hold. I have bad images of torrents rushing into the neighbor's yard. Talk about your water breaking.

DECEMBER 18

It's strange that now that we're only a week away from Christmas, I'm finding myself struggling to recall the certainty Maura and I have had all fall that we'd be feeling, anew and deeply, grief over Gail's death, that an overriding pain would sand the cheerful edge off the season. The sadness is certainly there, a complex mixture of gloom and helplessness. But the mood is not what I'd expected.

Maura and I talked long about this today in the kitchen, while we were cooking. She's sad, she says, but not unhappy. To the surprise of both of us, the simple reality of being pregnant makes this Christmas feel better than last year's, which was gloomy because of the miscarriages. And, to be honest, the days last Christmas that we spent in Vermont at Gail's house weren't all eggnog-ishly relaxing. There was a quiet tension between Gail and Maura that made everyone uncomfortable. No one talked anything out. I don't claim to understand the details, though it seems a version of what happens between so many parents and grown children, and maybe was exacerbated by Gail living by herself way up there and being a bit possessive of Maura's attention. In any case, there is no such tension this year. There are other lousy things, but a friction between mother and daughter is not one of them.

God knows I've felt that kind of friction with my own parents, and have gotten brief tastes of it between me and Maeve — enough to let me know that Years One-through-Five aren't a reliable indicator of what'll happen in, say, Year Fourteen. Or in Year Forty. My parents, God bless them, are healthy and thriving. But I admit to a fascination with the idea of adopting a new identity, of no longer being the child.

"It's a trade-off," says Maura, when I ask her crassly how she feels about having that change forced upon her. "You give up continuity, a sense of connection to the past. And whatever your parents can still give you that you've always gotten from them."

This is probably my way of rationalizing the benefits of being an older parent. With luck, Maura and I'll be around long enough to get our kids to adulthood, but if we kick off then, maybe the advantages to them of getting to adopt new roles will outweigh the disadvantages. So all we have to do is make it till then—and then hope that, rather than die, we don't deteriorate into some drooling, shitting, helpless beings that they have to spend all their time taking care of.

DECEMBER 19

The other day, in the pile of Gail's files and small possessions that we've sort of hidden away in a closet upstairs, I came across the Christmas gifts she'd bought on her cruise: a book about the stained-glass windows in Canterbury Cathedral, a porcelain nameplate for Maeve from Ireland, two Christmas tree ornaments, an illustrated copy of *The Canterbury Tales*. There's something both eerie and comforting about having them here, and now we have to decide whether to wrap them as she would have, or simply let them flow quietly into the sea of other things in the house. (I'm sure we'll wrap Maeve's, at least.)

DECEMBER 20

Went to tour the Labor & Delivery floor of the hospital today. Despite the pinks and lavenders, it all seemed entirely medical. As Maura said afterwards, "It's nice to see it, but it does make everything seem more imminent." I got queasy as the nurse was showing us the birthing room and explaining how the bed adjusted, where the emergency supplies were, and how to use the birthing ball (appropriately shaped like a huge egg). We saw the neonatal intensive care unit. The whirlpool. The nurses' stations. The family waiting-room. It all seemed functional and capable. Nothing fancy. On the other hand, I liked the nurses very much, and the relaxed atmosphere of the floor. Our tour guide, Valerie, was laid-back and friendly, patient and articulate, answering any question we could think of, including my not-so-subtle one about what makes St. Joe's a Catholic hospital. I wanted to test the save-the-baby-before-the-mother waters. "We've got some crucifixes on the walls, is about it," she said. They deliver about two thousand babies a year in that hospital—"not so many that it's crazy all the time, but enough to keep us busy," she said.

While we were at the hospital, Maeve went to our friend Lib's house to decorate Christmas cookies with Lib's five-year-old nephew Nicholas, who lives in Australia and is visiting for a couple of weeks. I only had to hear him say "Maeve" once with his killer accent before I was bowled over, and I don't know how Maeve kept from falling in love. Plus, he's got engagingly floppy hair, a cute smile, and the ability and nonchalance to plop himself down onto the piano bench without warning and play "Jingle Bells."

"He takes piano lessons," Maeve told us.

When we got home, I said to Maura, "I think Curtis has competition."

"A piano-playing Australian is tough," she agreed.

But when Curtis came over in the afternoon for a play-date (a real boy day for Maeve), he brought her an elaborate ring box, which Maeve was thrilled with and into which she put her engagement ring *and* the engagement bracelet that Curtis also added to today's gift. It was a suave move on Curtis's part, though I couldn't quite make him understand why he didn't want to announce to Maeve—as he did—that he'd gotten both of them really cheap at a garage sale.

DECEMBER 22

Maura's bronchitis is pretty much gone, but she has only enough energy these days to walk ten minutes before having to sit down. She and I went to the mall yesterday to pick up a few things for Maeve, and we could've had Calvin with us for all the speed we achieved. We'd go into a toy store and begin consulting, and then she'd say she had to go sit down and I would look closely at board games for fifteen minutes until either she came back or I went out to ask her whether she thought Maeve was old enough for Yahtzee. Today, she's still wiped out from that trip.

DECEMBER 23

Man, the weather has changed. We're in an early-season thaw. Nearly all of the snow is melted, and yesterday it was actually fifty-five degrees. There's the usual rejoicing about this among people who assume that warmth is good no matter what, though I'm not one to join in on it. I look forlornly out the kitchen window and see that the ice that was on the rink — the top inch or so had frozen — is gone. Now it's a man-made pond. If temperatures don't take a dive again soon, I'll be sitting on the back steps with a shotgun to keep ducks from settling in. Alas, it's supposed to be above freezing for another week.

DECEMBER 24

At night, I get the bed to myself for hours at a time — a guilty pleasure ten years into a marriage. Maura's found the couch to be more comfortable, and so she has been moving out there by about 2:00 each night. Sometimes Maeve will pad in around 4:00 or 5:00, and I can let her stay rather than hefting her back to her own bed — another guilty pleasure.

But the guilt is not always tempered by any pleasure. This morning I lay under the covers wondering at my lack of ability to empathize fully with Maura's condition. I mean my own utter inability to understand what she's feeling right now. She was coughing, rolling around and trying to get into a comfortable position, and I lay there unable to think of anything except how cozy I was. It was cold outside the covers, and I was trying to concentrate on an interesting dream I was having about sharing some chewing tobacco with a German shopkeeper. But I was also really trying to make myself feel what Maura might be feeling, as her hacks and bouncing around intruded upon my contentment. The best I could do was think about, when I lay on my side, how my own belly felt softer and plumper from the Christmas cookies I've been snacking on the past few days. But I knew that was like the Callahan cartoon in which a thin but curvaceous woman comes upon a homeless man squatting on the sidewalk holding a handwritten sign that says "Food." The woman exclaims, "Food! That's my problem too!"

It strikes me a few times every hour that right now is the heart of Maura's pregnancy, that these last two weeks are crunch time, what it all comes down to. This is the real test, and if I miss it because I'm in my little cocoon of comfort, then I will have missed something vital.

What's frustrating is figuring out exactly what it is that I don't want to miss, because, as Nature and all the pregnancy magazines tell me: it's not my experience.

DECEMBER 25

Maeve has learned to whistle, by sucking in rather than blowing out. She's gotten admirably good at it, and every couple of minutes she'll whistle spontaneously, a short but powerful burst. It's like living with a bird.

Also, my sister gave her a digital watch for Christmas, and when she has it strapped to her wrist she announces the time every minute. It's wearing.

DECEMBER 26

Christmas has passed. It's two weeks until the due date, a span that has no meaning to me. I can't decide whether it's a kid's two weeks—that is, forever—or an adult's. In some ways I'm acting as if it's the former—still not getting around to taping the doctor's number on to the refrigerator, putting off a trip to Babies 'R' Us for that equipment (diaper bag, changing table pad, suction ball for stuffed nostrils) that has the distant familiarity of an old college textbook. I *used* to spend a lot of time with this stuff. It's impossible to imagine the drama that will soon descend upon us. We're living a lazy life right now, sleeping late, finishing breakfast at about 10:00, letting hours go by with no accomplishments besides taking the dog for a short walk. This is the way people live at the beach, at least old people like us. I probably ought to be worried that I'm not worried about doing more to prepare. It's the joke about having a leaky roof but not fixing it when it's raining because it's too wet and not fixing it when it's dry because it doesn't leak then.

Anyway, at this point most of my mental preparation, if you can call it that, is an emptying of mind. Can I imagine the physical problems that might occur with this baby, or do anything about them right now? No. I put it out of my head. Can I imagine what it's going to be like to be exhausted for months on end? No. I don't think about it. Can I predict and prepare for how this new kid is going to affect family dynamics, how his presence is going to change Maeve's life in ways she might resent? No. We'll deal with it when it comes. Can I design a defensive strategy against the years of hyperactivity and rambunctiousness that having a boy in the house is going to bring? (We visited Curtis and his family last night for some beer and apple pie, and Curtis was zooming around unpredictably like the remote-control car he got for Christmas. "They're not all like this," Lynniece said. "Maybe you'll get a quiet one." Mere politeness on her part.) Anyway, no. I silently await the challenges.

Maura is trying to prepare, at least, for the exhaustion. I suggested that maybe an early birth would be good, since we're not doing much else at the moment. We could go stock up on videos, but why not have a kid instead? "No," she said. "I need a week to rest. Nine o'clock bedtimes. Lots of sleep. Good food."

So I guess we're on heightened alert, the orange level in the Bush administration's color scheme of danger. I ignore nearly everything that comes out of the Bush White House, but the advice they give for living at the orange level seems appropriate in a useless kind of way. "Be vigilant, but live your lives normally." Next week it'll rise to the red level. I suppose we'll be even more vigilant, and I'll put the doctor's number on the fridge.

Right now, the most imminent danger remains a possible collapse of the ice rink. The low side of the yard continues to take the full weight of all of that water, and the extra brackets and stakes seem ridiculously puny, though they're holding so far. The boards in the danger zone are leaning outward about fifteen degrees off vertical. If it goes, I'm screwed. I doubt I'd rebuild. If it would just get and stay cold, the damn thing would freeze and stay where it is, or move only glacially.

DECEMBER 27

Here's a difference between old parents and young ones. My nephew Ryan has gotten his new daughter's name tattooed on his forearm. It's in big letters that look like Chinese characters. BAILEY. He showed it off when he went to my parents' house for Christmas dinner. My sister asked him what happens if he ends up having five or six kids. "I guess we'll give them short names," he said.

Maeve has decided—or she did at least briefly—that she wants to be a boy. She told this to Maura last night as Maura was putting her to bed.

"Oh? Why?" Maura asked, not all that happy to hear this Freudian turn of events, especially after all of the cheering about the power of the egg during Maura's dinner-time lecture last summer.

"Because boys are tough," Maeve said. "They can do anything they want. Curtis can do a lot more things outside than I can."

This is true, and I've worried about it off and on for the last couple of years, though Maeve's less developed athleticism has never seemed to bother her. She used to come home from preschool last year and say that they'd played freeze tag in gym class, and that when it was her turn to chase people, she never caught anyone. She said it matter-of-factly, without any hint of frustration. She seemed completely focused on the fun of the chase.

"Well, you know a lot of tough girls," Maura pointed out. "Lainie is tough."

"Yeah," Maeve agreed. "One time she punched me in the chest."

"Oh. Well, Esmé is tough."

"Yeah. But I'm not tough."

"*I* think you are. You were tough last week when you told some kids to give back the toys they'd taken from you."

This small reminder, Maura reported, seemed to turn things around. Words are Maeve's strength, and she was happy to have it pointed out that toughness could reside there just as much as in her body.

"Besides," Maura said, proceeding gently, knowing that Maeve also likes distinctions, "some kids are *only* tough, which makes them mean. You're tough and kind. That's a harder thing to be."

DECEMBER 28

It's 1:00 in the morning, and I've finished a new list of boys' names. Maura and I agreed to each come up with ten new ones, and then winnow it down from there. We've got six or seven baby-name books, and I've been through each of them, as well as the phone book, every novel and short story collection on our shelves that I like, memoirs, plays, poems. It all becomes nonsensical after a while, and it's like being introduced around at a party. Who can keep everyone straight?

I hope we can give him a name that he likes as much as Maeve likes hers. We got her a couple books last spring, when we were in Ireland, about the historical/mythological Queen Maeve, the toughie who probably punched people in the chest whenever she wanted.

We've exchanged lists. I'm looking at Maura's. We have three names in common. Others I've already crossed off, just as she's probably downstairs crossing off most of mine. That's okay. We've agreed to wait a few hours before telling each other what we think. I need at least that much time to stop thinking what I really am thinking, which is that since this is a boy, he's more mine to name than he is Maura's. Doesn't gender get me extra ownership here?

Give me a little while, and I'll come around to understanding—maybe even agreeing—that it doesn't.

I really don't see how she could have put some of these names on her list.

"There's nothing better than feeling cozy sheets and a soft bed," Maeve said tonight, "especially if you're blind."

We've been reading a book about Helen Keller.

DECEMBER 29

Well, I was reminded again today of how having either a boy or a girl leads you into its own separate world of unfairness, distortion, prejudice. Cheerful thoughts, I know. They came to me while I was reading an article in a pregnancy magazine while we waited in the doctor's office. The article was about how schools are unintentionally set up to facilitate boys' failures. Of course I'm as familiar as the next semiconscious American with the unfairnesses that girls face, and the battles that their parents ought to be ready to fight. But it's easier to think that a boy can slide right into the power structure and that the world is set up to lead him to success. Apparently, not so.

The article argued that the nerves in boys' fingers do not develop as quickly as those in girls' fingers, and so it's more difficult for the boys to handle a pen early on. Hence, they have trouble writing, and get frustrated by their lack of progress. Who knows whether this theory holds up at all? The five- and six-year-old boys I know seem to be able to write just as well as the five- and six-year-old girls.

Of course, in later school years, the tables turn, because boys get so aggressive that they demand the bulk of the attention, leaving the girls in the background.

The first thing this article made me think was, Great, now I get to fight both battles. But that's not such a bad thing, I suppose. If you have to fight one, isn't it better to know what's happening on the other side, too, so that you're a more informed fighter? People always say that it'll be good for Maeve to have a little brother. I think it might actually be good for me as the father of a daughter.

It's completely quiet in the house. Even Maeve seems to have burrowed herself into a cone of silence, playing with dolls and looking through books. I don't know what this hush portends, if anything, though it seems the right thing to have about us at the moment. I only worry about Maeve, and so we occasionally shuffle her off to a rambunctious friend's house, where she gets her fill and then comes back into the fold, into the sanctuary.

DECEMBER 30

Maura and I winnowed last night. We began by taking turns explaining our rationale for each of our ten choices. "It sounded interesting when I wrote it down," I found myself saying for several of them, then shrugging my shoulders and moving on. One name we both really liked but can only imagine giving to a dog. It got stricken from the list (though added to a list for future dogs). Still, we went slowly, methodically, giving each name a chance to rise up and surprise us. We lingered over some for a good while, rolling them around on our tongues, doing the thing where you say the name with different modulations. It's important that a name sounds good when you scream it in anger. By the time we each reduced our lists to three, we were in close but not perfect agreement. My top choice was in second place for her. This core of acceptability added a great comfort to the room, as if we'd knitted the baby three sweaters, one of which was bound to fit and keep him warm. We'll let it all mellow for a while.

DECEMBER 31

We're a week and a day from the due date, and tonight was the first time that I've heard that postpartum depression is more common for the second pregnancy than for the first, even if there wasn't a hint of it the first time around — which there wasn't for Maura. This news came from our friend Rita, who has five grown children. She said this very thing had happened to her — all bliss and ecstasy with Number One, then gloominess and misery with Number Two. The subject came up because Rita is giving me a book manuscript that her sister Patricia — our old friend who died of leukemia last summer — had left behind. Patricia had shopped it around a little, but then she got sick and had to give it up. I told Rita I'd read it and see whether we could do something with it. It's about Patricia's years of depression. "You can read it, but don't let Maura see it," Rita said. She also warned me that I'd better be prepared to take extra care of Maura in the months ahead.

I don't disregard this kind of information lightly, especially because Rita is one of those people who knows so much, who is incredibly in tune with the world and with herself, that I believe pretty much anything she says, especially because she delivers even ominous news like this with her charming smile.

I didn't know whether to mention this subject at all to Maura, or simply to prepare myself, or to squash it all down into the back of my brain where it won't gnarr and menace until I need it. If I ever do.

But then I remembered the story from Maura's family about her grandmother, who was supposedly suicidal after one of her births. I don't know which one. That uncertainty, plus my craving to be in the loop at this stage on as many angles of the pregnancy as possible, made me feel as if I had to tell Maura what Rita had said.

"Have you heard about this pattern?" I asked her.

"No," she said abruptly, "and I don't want to hear it."

JANUARY 1

The new year begins in warmth. Today I had to use the snow shovel to fish a dead squirrel out of the deep end of the rink. "Did you not see the NO SKATING sign?" I asked him. Maura suggested I leave him there, as a curiosity for the kids once the ice does freeze. He could be our mascot. The middle schoolers, though, would be chipping through the ice to get him so they could scare the little kids off the rink.

JANUARY 2

No year-end tax break for us, and no prizes and local fame that come with having the first baby of the new year. Another woman delivered at 12:04 a.m.—about as timely a birth as you can imagine, if you're in that race.

Anyway, things are steady. "I think I'm nesting," Maura said when I came home this afternoon. "I've cleaned out all my drawers." We set up a shelf for diapers and related paraphernalia. Atop of it we placed a little pillow that Maura's sister Jennifer crocheted. It says "Bebé." That's about as much decorating as we'll do, since the boy is going to be in our room with us for the first few months. There's really no place else to put him. His cradle will be at the foot of our bed, and when he graduates to the crib, maybe that'll go there, too, if there's room.

Maeve's old crib is in the attic, in parts. I hope I saved all the nuts and bolts. If not, I tell Maura, I'll take the rink apart and build something out of those two-by-twelves.

JANUARY 3

This morning I took Maeve to a "Sibling Class" at St. Joe's. The nurse, Christine, showed the soon-to-be older sisters (there were no boys there) how to hold a baby, how to swaddle it, what not to feed it (French fries, carrots, ice cream, bubble gum), what to do if they're feeling left out (tell Mom and Dad), what to do if they get annoyed at the baby (go outside and run it off). It was a sweet presentation. Maeve fine-tuned her baby-holding technique. I learned that baby powder is now as dangerous as lead dust (can be breathed in and cause pneumonia). We had a little birthday party for the kids-to-be, with cake that made my throat tickle, even though it was well before lunchtime.

Right in the middle of the class, a bell rang gently.

"Do you know what that is?" Christine asked. No one did. "A new baby was just born here." They ring the bell every time. It's like being inside *It's a Wonderful Life*.

All of the parents, of course, were old hands at having a kid, though I couldn't help wishing there were other kinds of classes some parents would sign up for. One father in particular. He was a cheerful guy in his early thirties, and he was there with his wife and nine-year-old daughter. After about three minutes, I wanted to take him aside and lecture him on how to raise a girl. Every comment he made to her was a tease, a mocking—all done in the spirit of fun, of course. It was all small stuff, insignificant in tiny doses. When Christine mentioned that the kids were going to be making sock dolls for the new babies, the father said to his daughter, "I hope they don't smell like your socks." When Christine asked whether any of the kids had pets, the father made a wisecrack about his daughter bringing home every turtle and hamster she could find. Small pokes. His wife laughed at every one of them, and the daughter grimaced gamely at most, but not all. Sometimes she stiffened. I wanted to tell the guy: *Observe* the reaction. Save the wittiness for your drinking buddies, who will either tell you to shut up or give you their own right back. Continue to talk to your daughter this way and you'll find yourself having no significant conversations with her at all in a few years when she's ready to give as good as she gets.

The guy and his wife are having a son this spring. I wouldn't put *all* my money on the chances that he doesn't tease his son so much, but I'd bet most of it.

It's going to be so hard to raise a boy who will let himself be ruled by empathy rather than ego.

We're three days into January, and still the warmth lingers on. Fifty-five today. We drove out to a nature center for Curtis's birthday party, and the plan had been for the kids to go snowshoeing through the woods. That's what they did last year, in a fairly brutal blizzard. This year, they all simply took a walk on the bare trails, in sneakers.

Tomorrow night, things are supposed to change. They say we'll get a real blast, and it'll be around ten every night for a week. This is wonderful news from the point of view of a rink maker. It makes me think that people who don't like the cold simply don't have enough personal reasons for it to *be* cold. Everyone should have more of a stake in there being ice and snow and winds that whip right through even the bulkiest sheepskin coats.

I've got my fingers crossed, too, that it'll be bitter cold when the baby is born. Let's say, oh, ten below. And throw in some snow. Double-digits worth, coming down in gigantic flakes so fast that it'll be like being in the line of fire of a snowblower. I'm not masochistic. I simply want *context*. A story. I hated it at the time, but after it was over I really liked the fact that it was 104 degrees in Little Rock on the day Maeve was born. It stayed so hot that two days later the flowers people had sent didn't even survive the thirty-mile drive home. They came out of the hospital and immediately wilted. I don't know how Maeve survived it.

Gail had been down in Arkansas then, and when Maura's contractions got close enough, I drove us all on a back road at about eighty, Gail in the passenger seat with a watch and a yellow pad of paper on which she was writing the time of each contraction, Maura in the back in pain. It was exciting, especially after the dullness of waiting around for a week or two.

"The only thing that would make this better," I said to them, "would be to get pulled over." And at that instant a trooper crested the hill in front of us, and then quickly turned around and hit the lights. When he walked up to the car, I got to say the classic words: "My wife's in labor. We're on our way to the hospital."

Gail leaned over and showed him her paper. He leaned down and looked at Maura. Then he stepped back, clearly not wanting to be anywhere in our vicinity. He didn't offer to escort us. All he said was, "Well, put your flashers on." And I cranked it back up to eighty.

There is nothing on the agenda but to have a baby. Maura seemed to realize this tonight, and she went into something of a meditative state, sitting quietly in the digesting chair and not saying much at all. After a while I asked her, "Are you ready?"

"Yeah, I guess I am," she said softly, sounding surprised at the way the feeling had come on so suddenly.

We wait.

My parents were going to drive up from Ohio on Monday, but I called them and told them to stay put until something happens.

JANUARY 5

Maura's doctor likes to tell us that our fears are relics of "the old days"—outdated notions about which we need not worry ourselves here in the twenty-first century. "Well, in the old days, yeah," he'll say with a dismissive chortle. And we'll feel as if we got our ideas about pregnancy and childbirth when we were in our teens and twenties, and that we've clung blindly to them, refusing to keep up with the latest research—like someone who memorized the periodic table in 1965 and can't accommodate the new elements discovered since then. I bet he never uses the "old days" line with his twenty-one-year-old patients. Maura asked him today about inducing, and the fact that she'd heard that one of the dangers of inducing for a VBAC is that you go from zero to sixty in about three seconds.

"Well, in the old days, yeah," he said. "Back then, they'd either give you an injection or they'd have you snort it. So you got this big dose, and then whatever happened, happened. We haven't done that in *years*—certainly since before I started. *I've* never done it. Now we give it through an IV, and we can give whatever we need to, based on the woman's reactions. We adjust it so that we can bring on a normal labor pattern."

To hear some doctors tell it, medicine has an answer for everything. I remain suspicious.

Medicine certainly doesn't have an answer for the question of this week, which is, as my friend Mike put it: What to do with that little swath of skin? Or I should say that medicine has a very *definite* answer, but that it's the exact opposite of the answer medicine had just a few years ago. On this issue, it turns out, I really was operating on the old periodic table. The last I heard, circumcision was a *good* thing—except, of course, for the possible psychological trauma and just the idea of the barbaric procedure. But medically, yes, very good. I revealed my squareness when I asked the doctor if we had to sign a form or something in order to get this kid circumcised. He almost rolled his eyes at me.

"Well, if you want that, I have to give you the spiel first," he said.

"We *do* want it," I said, immediately defensive, and really having no idea whether Maura was part of this "we." Somehow, we hadn't yet talked about circumcision. "But give the spiel."

"Now, in the old days," he began, "they thought that circumcision reduced the risk of penile cancer and also cervical cancer for the woman. They thought it was probably generally healthier all around. Today, everyone agrees that it's purely cosmetic surgery. No medical benefit. So if you want to get rid of your wrinkles, or get your breasts enlarged, or get rid of your spare tire, it's cosmetic surgery, just like circumcision. We're the only country in the world that does this as a matter of routine. If you're Jewish, you do it because the religion says to. Otherwise, cosmetic."

It wasn't a spiel I really wanted to hear, I realized once I'd heard it. I think the doctor could tell he'd thrown me into another uncertainty.

"I'm not going to tease you if you really want it done," he promised. "But, you know, we used to take tonsils out regularly. Now we leave them in because they keep kids healthy."

I sighed. "Well, how many do you do, percentage-wise?"

"It's fifty-fifty," he said.

When I talked to Mike later in the day, he pointed out, "You know, the King was whole. So at least I've read in a couple of biographies." Mike is the one who pointed out to us last summer that January 8 is like Christmas Day for the Presleytarians.

"If he's actually born on Elvis's birthday," I told him, "we'll take that into consideration."

"I'm going to turn this one over to you," Maura said, when I was rolling around the doctor's argument in my mind, resenting him for puncturing our recent blissed-out mindlessness. "You're the guy, and, you know, I'm happy with either way."

"So now it's up to me to decide to torture him for no good reason?" I said.

"Dear, it's not torture," she said gently. "He's not going to remember it any more than you remember your own circumcision." Then she added, "But if he *is* circumcised, all I ask is that you change the bandages while he's healing."

I spent way too long after that looking at very disturbing and graphic anti-circumcision web sites, meant to make me feel like someone who was only half a step away from holding lit cigarettes against my baby's skin.

Snow. A couple of inches each of the previous two days. And the cold that should've been here weeks ago. I closed all of the windows yesterday, and with the ferocity of this cold front, I expect they'll stay closed for a good long time. Till April, probably.

january 6

I just finished a very scientific survey on the state of the young penises in our neighborhood. I asked the moms at the bus stop, as we bounced lightly in the newly arrived cold, what they did with *their* sons. The sample was smallish, since there were only two moms there, but there was unanimity between them. Both put their sons under the knife. On the other hand, they both have sisters who *didn't*. Expanding out for the secondary data, we're at a tie. The fifty-fifty that Maura's doctor quoted us.

One of the moms, Lisa, is a nurse, and she confirmed what the doctor had said: circumcision is not a medical issue. But Lynniece chimed in with the information that her uncircumcised nephew has had problems with urinary tract infections.

"Ten years ago, there was a real push for it," Lisa said. "But now we've swung back to the other end of the pendulum."

"It's like religion," I said. "You decide, based on something completely arbitrary, that you're going to take a certain path."

"And in twenty years," Lisa said, "your son will say, 'Dad, you ruined my life!'"

"And you don't know which choice now will bring on that damage!" I cried.

Lynniece left us with what I wish was more of a ringing endorsement. "I would do it," she said, "as long as they do a good job."

When I ask other people for their opinions on circumcision, lots of them mention that the boy might be more comfortable if he's like me.

"Believe me," I tell them, "he'll be like me in more ways than he wants to."

JANUARY 7

Just before waking up this morning, I had a dream that Maeve had died. It's not clear how, and it didn't matter. The odd thing was that she was simply gone, and I had no words to articulate that. In the dream, I talked with friends on the phone, and I didn't even mention that Maeve was dead. They didn't know. I was in a sunny room, and after I hung up the phone, I slumped in a corner among the dust balls and the clumps of dog hair, and I whimpered. Then I heard Maeve in the kitchen, yelling about having to brush her teeth, and I woke up. A lousy way to start the day.

This is an easy one to decipher. The danger of Maeve being wiped out by the appearance of the new kid.

Maura's on the ball with this. She's realized that we need to buy Maeve a present when the baby's born, to keep her in the loop.

First, though, Maura has to buy a new toiletries bag. She's at the mall right now looking for one. She's had her present one for years, but now says she'd be ashamed to show up at the hospital with it. It seems just the tiniest bit irrational to me, especially since she had to go out in the snow and cold for this one thing, but as Jennifer said when I talked to her a few minutes ago, "At this point, whatever's good for the pregnant woman is good for everyone."

It's the evening before Maura's official due date, and it's shaping up to be a classic night to have a baby: heavy snow, high winds, a frigid temperature, and a wind chill well below zero. The roads are slick, and the plows will be out soon, rumbling down the street and beginning their usual task of blocking us in at the end of the driveway. I took Calvin for a walk just to the corner two hours ago, and the snow was beginning to be heavy enough so that when he got back into the kitchen his head and back were covered fully with white. On the pre-bedtime walk we just took, so he could have one last squirt, there were three new inches of snow.

Gail left us her Subaru, with its all-wheel drive and its big, grippy tires. I think about her — and silently thank her — each time we take it out in the snow, but I will do so even more fervently if the trip to the hospital is as I suspect it might be.

JANUARY 8

At the doctor's office today, on this day that's loomed in our consciousnesses since last summer, the nurse hooked Maura up to a monitor for what she called a non-stress test — which, I guess, doesn't require the baby or Maura to get on a treadmill. Maura sat very still, and for twenty minutes we listened to the baby's heartbeat pound loudly through the small exam room, watched two needles on the machine squiggle their way up the roll of shiny paper. "Did you feel that contraction?" the nurse asked Maura. The second needle had recorded a big sweeping curve in the middle of a relatively straight line. "No," Maura said. You would've thought she had to feel it, though I suppose there is much that happens in our guts to which we're blessedly oblivious. The nurse brought Maura cookies, and then remembered me just as she was walking out the door. "Would you like some too?" I said yes. Most of the time when I accompany Maura on these visits I feel like one of those red lights on top of a radio tower that glows bright for a second and then fades back to darkness, with the dark periods longer than the illuminated ones. Maura's light glows constantly, and she gets everyone's undivided attention. That was certainly true this morning in the waiting area, where she had great status among the other women because she'd gone the distance, she was *there*.

"I've been lying in bed awake at night thinking about you," her doctor said when he came in.

"I lie awake and think about myself, too," Maura said.

He proclaimed the graph wonderful, then checked for dilation but didn't find any.

Maura tried to feign patience through pursed lips.

"We're only at the due date," the doctor said comfortingly. "We're in great shape. What I propose we do is wait, and you should feel free to go into labor anytime. Otherwise, come back on Monday, and we'll see what's what." He raised his palms to indicate that we were all in agreement.

"Wait how long?" Maura asked.

Doctors like to keep you in the here and now, get you thinking about how things can work themselves out naturally before you get to a crisis point. I think half of a good doctor's job is keeping people calm. I could forgive some sizeable gaps in medical knowledge if my doctor is, say, someone who might record relaxation tapes on the side to supplement his income. "If it comes to it, I'll let you go until next Thursday," he told Maura soothingly, as if he were telling her she could have an extra few days to finish a homework assignment. "There's nothing dangerous about going a week over." And then without changing the calming tone of his voice, he told us, because he knows by now that we want to know whatever he knows, that things *can* get dicey if you go beyond forty-one — what with the fact that the placenta has its own lifespan and can shut down with little notice. Why build an organ that will last longer than it needs to? "After forty-one weeks the death rate for the baby goes up significantly," said our good doctor in a way that, surprisingly, didn't make us worry about the death of the baby. "After forty-two weeks, it goes up dramatically."

The store's closing, little dude. Please bring your final purchases to the register.

JANUARY 9

One day after the due date. The little guy's in there reading the newspaper. I already like him better because he didn't fall for something so trite as being born on Elvis's birthday. He'll have taste and subtlety.

I have to say that if I were him, I'd be in no great rush. It's supposed to be twenty below zero tonight — the kind of cold that freezes the hair inside your nostrils. Or, if you're like twelve hours old, the kind of cold that would numb you so much that you wouldn't know what kind of barbaric procedure someone was performing on you.

Which reminds me that I've made a decision on the circumcision. It ain't gonna happen. The kid's spared. This is such a load off of my mind. I can only imagine what he's thinking.

I don't know when I finally decided — probably during one of those blissed-out moments while standing in the bitter cold in the backyard, watching water freeze, when it was clear that Nature in all its ethereal glory is wonderful if you don't try to control it too much, if you simply feel the energy and the love and the karma, one of those lucid moments during which it was utterly comprehensible and oh so obvious that extra knives and procedures are just going to complicate everything — like buying an extended warranty on a car. Who needs it?

And I thought, This is what the kid will be. He'll be his own self, with his own little foreskin — an organic and well-adjusted human being. He'll be . . . whole.

I tried to start the old car a little while ago, but it's frozen up solid. So it's an extra good thing that Gail's car is here, though that one gave us its own trouble this morning when Maura and I went out to breakfast. It got us to the restaurant fine but wouldn't start afterwards. We warmed ourselves in a nearby bookstore and called Lynniece to come get Maura, so she could be home when Maeve's bus got there, but then a few minutes later I tried the car again and it roared immediately to life. It was a few degrees above zero at the time. If we need to go to the hospital tonight and the car doesn't start, I'm calling my buddies at the fire station. We'll have them chauffeur us in the ambulance.

Even with the cold, though, and even with my occasional moments of winter-induced bliss, I have great and painful doubts about the ice rink. I think I may be completely screwed with it. It's still got eight or ten inches of water under the ice, at the deepest point, and even though I check a half dozen times a day, I don't see much progress. There's a little opening in the boards at that corner where I can feel the plastic and measure the thickness of the ice — about six or seven inches right now. My only hope is that the frigid weather hangs on for four or five days. It's supposed to.

It all distresses me, because I don't see any likely way to solve the problem now. My first mistake was building the frame with such a variation in elevation. I can't do anything about that until the spring, when I plan to get a bulldozer in there to level everything. But I realize now that I could have been more patient, could have waited until it was really cold to put any water in, and then built the ice up in thin layers, a few inches at a time. Who knows, though? If I'd done that maybe the rink wouldn't have been ready until June.

So I can wait, or I can take a drastic measure that tempts me so much. I could punch a small hole in the bottom of the plastic, and let all that uncooperative water flow out. If all went right, the frozen slab would settle gently to the bottom of the rink, sealing the hole with its weight, and I could build up layers on top of it. But it's an all-or-nothing measure. If it didn't go right — about a ninety-nine-percent likelihood — the slab would crash downwards, ripping the plastic all around the rink into shreds, and for the next two months I'd have to look at a slanted and broken hunk of ice that resembles an especially tricky section for climbers on the face of Mt. Everest.

Patience.

I look at Maura and have only one question: Any contractions yet? I'm about as single-minded as Calvin, looking at me and asking: Any food you don't want? I think Maura wants to talk about other things, but then at other times she seems as trapped by the anticipation as I am.

The cold is making it so that most things don't work right, including the dog. Though he doesn't go out much on days like this, his back hips seem to be worse, and he lurches around the house bumping into things, sometimes having his back legs collapse altogether. Maura mentioned today the idea of "not prolonging his discomfort," but the idea makes me queasy and distressed—not only for Calvin's sake but because it recalls all too vividly the decision Maura and Jennifer had to make only months ago about their mother. I've never had to make a decision like that for a pet. We didn't have pets when I was growing up, and the cats I've had since have gone on peacefully of their own accord. Calvin makes no complaints about any pain he might be in. The only emotion he seems to show is embarrassment over falling down. Otherwise, he's fine.

JANUARY 10

The next day, and an utterly traumatic one for Calvin. When Maura, Maeve, and I came back from a trip to the grocery store, we found him in the bedroom, unable to get up. His back legs were under the bed—there's about an eight-inch clearance that he somehow works himself into often, though usually it's his head, so that when he begins to get up he cracks his skull on the underside of the wooden bed frame. This time he couldn't drag himself out from under there in order to stand. He has no scooting ability. He must've been there for a couple of hours, whining and struggling. By the time we found him, he'd quit whining, but he was shaking terribly. He'd shit and pissed on himself. I pulled him out, and he couldn't stand up, from being so shaken. He leaned against me, and I spoke softly to him, though he probably can't hear any soft voices, and I held him and scratched him. Maura cleaned up the mess.

I carried him out to the kitchen so he could drink some water, but he either didn't want any or simply couldn't get his breath enough to try. He was breathing fast and shallow, and every part of him continued to shake. For an hour I supported him—it seemed he wanted to be on his feet—and we tried to brush out the clump of shit on his hindquarters and kept petting him. For a while he lay on his belly with his back legs splayed in odd directions, and I fed him Scooby Snacks, which he ate with the focused obsession with which I eat cookies when I'm upset. Maura cried and then called a friend to get a recommendation on a vet, and simply to talk to someone else to ease her anguish.

If a vet were easily available — if it weren't late Saturday afternoon, if we'd already taken Calvin to a vet here in Syracuse — I don't know what might have happened. He seemed to have taken an irreversible dive.

Finally, though, I took him outside, hoping the cold air would calm him down. It seemed to help. He stood warily, eating snow, and after a while was able to take a few steps around the patio. I carried him back inside — it was freezing out there — and gave him two aspirin wrapped in sliced ham. Slowly, he got his breath back, and the shaking stopped. He began to stand with his previous uncertainty, which was at least a big improvement. He hobbled back into the bedroom and, after a painful couple of minutes of circling his spot, let himself fall to the rug. He went to sleep almost immediately. When I checked on him a little later, he looked like he always does, calm enough to be dead.

The poor, poor guy.

JANUARY 11

Calvin and the baby are suddenly and so definitely on those converging paths that I had imagined early in the fall — the baby coming towards birth and the dog going towards death. Suddenly, within the last twenty-four hours, it looks inevitable that they each will cross the boundary at just about the same time.

It's Sunday, and Calvin has been distressed for hours, walking around the house as if he's forgotten something important. It's almost a panic. He goes in circles, always clockwise, and sometimes his back legs cross over each other and send him tumbling sideways. It's nearly too painful to watch.

"It's only going to get worse," Maura finally said, an oblique statement of the kind we've been warily trying out. All weekend neither of us has come right out and spoken of putting the dog down — even yesterday in the worst moments. But we've both been thinking of little else.

"Call Jennifer and talk it out with her," I urged Maura.

And so she did, and a half hour later she came back into the kitchen and handed the phone silently to me. She was crying.

Jennifer was calm on the other end of the line, able to provide some objectivity from the Illinois flatlands. I told her again what Maura had certainly already told her—about Calvin being trapped under the bed yesterday, about the way Calvin was pacing crookedly with a look of alarm or dread in his eyes, about the charged air in which we were all living. I told her there didn't seem to be any doubt about what ought to be done.

She agreed, and I could hear her begin to cry. There was a long silence while I let my throat loosen up. "If Mom were here, she would do it," Jennifer said.

"Do you think so?"

"Definitely."

"She did tell us to use our discretion," I said.

"This would be the time for that," said Jennifer.

After we hung up, I gave Calvin another piece of ham. I slipped him four or five Scooby Snacks. And then a few more. There was half a box to get through.

JANUARY 12

Monday. In the morning another trip to Maura's doctor's office. We're to the point at which the nurses express sympathy, as if we found out right at the end that we need one or two more credits to graduate. We shrug and go through the routine.

Another non-stress test. I watched the paper feed out of the machine, the needle zipping back and forth as the heartbeat shot up to 175 and then back down to 125, and ranged all over in between. It worried the hell out of me, until the doctor came in and looked at it and said, "What a healthy kid!" Everything still looks fine, except that the cervix refuses to dilate. "It's softer than it was last week," the doctor said, "and that's good." Even though she couldn't feel them, the monitor showed that Maura was having contractions every eight minutes. "Perhaps this is the precursor to real labor," said the doctor. The guy is eternally optimistic. I've grown to depend on that.

Maura's inner ear is red and inflamed, she can't hear out of it, and the doc's advice was to drink hot liquids and use some steam to try to unblock it. She's already had two blasts of antibiotics in the last month, because of the bronchitis, and he didn't want to throw more at her, in case she starts building up immunities to it.

So, home again, with another appointment for Thursday.

In the afternoon, it was off to the vet—a more apprehensive trip. In the morning, while I was cleaning up Calvin's pee from the living room floor, I'd said meanly to him, "This is the last time you'll do this, dog." But it turns out that it's probably not. Against what both Maura and I were sure of yesterday, we brought him back home with us.

Maybe it was the warmer weather—it reached thirty-five today—but Calvin had his old spunk back. Back from the edge of death. He was relatively calm, with only the normal number of falls.

We took him to a clinic recommended to us by some friends. All the vets and other staff there are women. Whether or not the gender homogeneity has anything to do with it, the place was welcoming and comfortable, with an aura of sympathy exuding from the receptionist, the vet herself, and even the young assistant whose job it is to hold the pets while the vet gives them shots or cleans their ears. There are glass jars of dog snacks placed conveniently around the office, like bowls of potato chips at a party. We had to drive all the way across town to get to the place, but it was worth it.

In the exam room, Calvin walked around and around in circles, the same thing he does at the dinner table each night, though there with no chair or human legs to get in his way. We each reached down and let our fingers run through his fur as he went by, so that it was almost like riding in a small boat, with our hands dangling over the side and being splashed every few seconds by gentle waves. Habits like this of Calvin's have come to be so expected that Maura and I were both surprised when the vet said that the obsessive circling is probably a sign that Calvin's had a stroke of some sort, evidence complemented by the way he tilts his head. "He's probably not all there mentally," she said.

Of course we felt both sad and relieved—the first because of the cruel similarity to his real owner's sickness, and the second because we're always happy about the blessed ignorance of those in pain.

The vet saw other signs: that Calvin's liver was probably giving out, that his kidneys are likely at the ends of their useful lives (he drinks obsessively, taking breaks only to walk in circles).

"I don't think we're talking about more than a matter of a few weeks," she said. "It could be longer, or shorter. But at this stage, there are really no medical measures that would be of any real help. Some buffered aspirin, like you've been doing, to take the edge off of any pain he might be feeling."

We all stood quiet for a minute. "Some people prefer to put an animal to sleep when it's still feeling pretty good," the vet continued, "as a way of letting it avoid the worst of the pain. I can give you a few minutes alone to talk about it."

"Oh, no," Maura said, as if she'd been caught off guard. "I can't do this today."

And I had to agree with her. Even with the expert evaluation of greater direness than we had assumed, Calvin was too perky. Faced with the very offer we'd probably have accepted yesterday or the day before, we suddenly weren't in the proper mental state, whatever that might be. I can't imagine what it'll take to get us there again, except for Calvin spiraling down precipitously.

The receptionist was genuinely happy to see Calvin come out of the exam room alive. I gave him a handful of snacks from her desk.

And so we lifted him into the back of the car and drove home. I watched him in the rearview mirror, and I drove gently. He was lurching left and right because he refused to lie down.

In between today's visits to medical clinics, I drove out to the country to get a cradle. Lynniece and Tim are lending us theirs, since their daughter has recently outgrown it, but the thing was at a little cabin Tim built on some land they'd bought last summer out by a tiny airport with a grass runway. Tim's a pilot. I drove as close to the cabin as I could, but there was too much snow on the runway to risk getting stuck out there, so I hiked the quarter-mile, with Maeve's plastic sled in hand. I got the cradle and put it on the sled and dragged it back. It was snowing heavily, the wind was blowing, and I felt like some pioneer bringing furniture to a new settlement. If I'd had a lantern, I would've been Michael Landon in *Little House on the Prairie*. I like this idea of working to get something so essential. It was, for a few minutes, almost as if I were building the thing myself.

JANUARY 13

When people see that Maura is still pregnant, they say, "Oh, you poor thing." It's actually the same thing that people are saying to Calvin these days when they see him.

JANUARY 14

If anyone ever made a movie of our glamorous lives, God knows there'd be a lot of editing required. There's a ton just in keeping this journal. I try to write down the drama of the experience, but most of what consumes us now is the struggle to wait. It doesn't make for good on-screen presentation. Maybe in a surreal art-house film, but maybe not even that.

We *could* speed things up, cut right to the chase, what with the knife waiting there for Maura and the needle for Calvin. Perhaps more pragmatic people would've already done that. Instead, we sit captive to our rationalizations — such as that Maura already knows how long it takes to recover from a C-section, and that there's a chance we could avoid that road this time.

With the dog, though, the week goes on and it becomes less clear why we're waiting, or what for. A "natural" death? A miraculous recovery? Even in our current muddled states of mind, I don't think either of us believes that the first is absolutely necessary or that the second is even within the realm of possibility. Calvin continues to stumble painfully (at least for us) around the house, continues to walk obsessively in clockwise circles in the kitchen every evening, continues to clonk his head loudly against the floor when he tries to stand or lie down and against the table legs and kitchen cabinets when he makes blind turns. For the last two mornings he's peed in the house before I could get him outside, even though we headed straight from bed to the back door. He's also quit finishing his dinner — last night eating only about a third of it. He's pure bones and fur. The fur is thick and starting to get matted, and I brush him out the best I can, but he could use a haircut and a shampoo. I had him scheduled for one for next Monday, but I called today to cancel it. "I'm not sure he'll even *make* it to Monday," I told the woman who runs the shop. "And even if he does, the vet says the grooming would be too much stress for him."

If we didn't have *both* of these things to wait for, I think we could let Calvin go on for weeks, if only from our own inertia. Also, killing something at this very moment — mercifully or not — seems like bad juju.

Still, the imminent birth forces us occasionally into some semblance of practical thinking. Maura pushes me to say when I think would be a good time for the inevitable trip back to the vet. I tell her I want to hold off a little.

"I kind of like the idea of overlap," I say. "Having Calvin and the baby alive in the world at the same time."

"I kind of like the idea of *no* overlap," she says. "Cleanliness."

No moves yet. Tomorrow, at forty-one weeks, we go see what the doc says. Then maybe other decisions will flow from that.

If there are miracles occurring around here, not the least amazing is that the rink is still standing, and that the ice is thickening. At the very bottom of the rink is maybe an inch of unfrozen water. And it is simply bitter, bitter cold out. This morning's paper pointed out that yesterday's high temperature in Syracuse was lower than the high temperature yesterday on Mars. It was only three-below here. It got up to twelve on Mars. Our low was eighteen-below.

I let water run onto the rink yesterday for four hours, adding another inch to the thickness, and the surface is smooth. Tonight, it'll be fifteen-below again.

After a slow and bundled walk around the block this evening, Maura said to me flatly, "There is really nothing more to talk about. People look at me, and they look sympathetic, but there is nothing more to say. I want to have the baby."

My parents have been here for several days now, having decided to make the drive even before anything happened. Maura's feeling the pressure of an audience, admitting that she's tempted to go have a C-section just so she doesn't keep all these people waiting. It's true that everyone isn't doing much besides hanging around in anticipation, like an army massed on the border for an invasion that keeps getting delayed by negotiations. There's the same kind of effort to keep up readiness and focus. My mother keeps saying, "Maybe it'll happen today." But I think she's the only one who believes it, or the only one who feels responsible for undertaking the pep talk. She says it with admirable optimism, anyway.

My father sits at the kitchen table and does crossword puzzles. He and I and my mom have gone through a lot of wine. Maeve plays with her dolls.

JANUARY 15

Once again, this morning, the monitor strapped onto Maura's tight belly. Two contractions in twenty minutes. She didn't feel either. Then the doctor checked her cervix. Afterwards, he took several steps backwards towards the wall.

"I'm moving out of hitting distance," he said.

"Nothing?" Maura asked.

"Nope."

Maura pursed her lips. After a few seconds, she said what she had said to me last night: "I want to have a baby."

The doctor nodded, but he clearly wanted to be careful, empathetic. "You say that with hesitation," he said, "as if you think I might be disappointed in you."

"No, not at all."

"Let me ask it this way," he said. "Some women want VBAC because they believe it'll make them feel more complete. Is that why you tried?" And just like that, he'd easily slipped into the past tense, the attempt to go natural already a memory. Maura was no longer trying, but had tried. She didn't correct him.

"No, not at all," Maura repeated.

"Or some women, like in Brazil, want the C-section so they can keep their vaginas like those of eighteen-year-olds."

"That's not it either," Maura said. "I really just want to have the baby."

"Okay," he said. "Let's have the baby. What are you doing tomorrow morning?"

"Tell me where to be, and I'll be there," said Maura.

"St Joe's. Nine o'clock. I'll tell them to expect you."

I had been keeping quiet, letting the conversation be completely between Maura and her doctor. But then I was included, as, oddly, everyone shook hands.

JANUARY 16

Deep, dense cloud cover, heavy snow, blowing winds, temperature just a few degrees above zero. This morning when we got up, it was almost exactly one hundred degrees colder than the day Maeve was born. Maura and I got our showers and got dressed. I ate breakfast, and Maura didn't because she was heading into surgery. It felt as if we were getting ready to go anywhere — to school, to the mall, to church. There were no cramps or contractions to color the actions, to give urgency. Only the wintry weather, the scraping of snow and ice off the car windows, the squeak of tires over the snow in the driveway, the two wrecks we passed along the way, the feeling of apprehension mixed with relief filling the cold car.

My parents stayed home with Maeve. They'd meet us there later.

At Labor and Delivery, a nurse gave Maura papers to sign, and then once she was in a bed, the supporting actors started showing up: a nurse to stick Maura for an IV, an aide to strap the monitor across her belly, another nurse to take vitals, the anesthesiologist to explain the dessert tray of drug choices. Maura was as uncomfortable as she'd been all week, truly heavy laden. I kept moving from one side of the bed to the other, trying to stay out of the nurses' ways. *They* kept moving from one side of the bed to the other to do some new task.

When the doctor popped in to say hello, he didn't look to me like anyone qualified to perform abdominal surgery — especially since, I realized, I'd never seen him with anything more dangerous than a stethoscope. "Speculum," Maura said when I whispered my doubt to her after he'd gone. Still, the nurses acted as if the doctor knew what he was doing. I gave myself over to the power of the institution.

They wheeled Maura down to the O.R., and I stood in the hallway, near a sign that said ABSOLUTELY NO CASUAL OBSERVATION. The O.R. actually had a big picture window, and I was very uncasually looking at Maura leaning forward with her head on the shoulder of a nurse. I thought for several minutes that she was crying, but the nurse was standing straight up, without her arms around Maura, as if she were trying to ignore her. The doctors and other nurses were mingling off to the side, laughing silently behind the glass. I couldn't make any sense of it, until I finally caught sight of the covered head of the anesthesiologist bent down close to Maura's back. Of course he was inserting his needle.

When they finally let me in, Maura was lying on the table, her arms out to her sides (I'd forgotten this disturbing detail from the last time). There was a blue towel rising above her chest, and the doctor and his assistant were already at work on the other side, prepping Maura's belly with yellow antiseptic. The anesthesiologist offered me a chair right next to Maura's head, but I stood, for the view.

Maura smiled, apparently only the tiniest bit loopy from the drugs and her complete immobility.

And then they began cutting. It was a quick zip, zap, and the doctor yanked around skin and muscle, worming his hands into the glop as if he were boning a chicken. Maura was staring intently at me, and so I had to keep looking mostly at her and only a little at the more dramatic scene with the doctors. I didn't find out until later that she wanted me to look at her so she could watch the action through the reflection in my glasses.

And then they pulled him out, a vernix-covered giant. He stretched on and on, and he had no wrinkles, as if the skin were pulled to exactly the right tension over his big bones and muscles. The doctor lifted him up over the blue wall so that Maura could see, and blood and amniotic fluid were dripping all over her face, into her eyes. I stuck out my hand to protect her, and I announced that she was getting soaked. "Oh she's a mother, she can handle it," the doctor said, laughing.

The nurse took the boy—with all of his toes and legs and fingers and ears and everything thing else apparently normal—to the other side of the room and laid him on the scale. Nine pounds, eleven ounces. As Jennifer said when we called to tell her later, "Holy shit." He is twenty-one inches long.

We have named him Fergus. A name from Irish royalty, just as Maeve is. Fergus Joseph. I like the name because it is manly, vigorous, soft at its beginning, punchy at its end. Some people are already calling him Gus.

I spent all day at the hospital, holding Fergus up in Maeve's lap, taking pictures, relearning how to swaddle a baby, helping see Maura through a rough few hours after the surgery, when her blood pressure dropped so that she would nearly faint if she sat up. She was racked by chills that even blankets warm from the dryer couldn't stop. The doctor seemed much more concerned about this condition than he had about the surgery itself, and he came back to the room every few minutes to see how she was doing. I refused to have any visions of horrible scenarios, and I put my trust once again completely in the doctor, who patiently worked whatever magic he had, and eventually got the blood pressure back up, got rid of the fever, and got some food into Maura's stomach. Then she sat there happily, the plastic balloons on her legs inflating and deflating every thirty seconds, to make sure she didn't get any blood clots.

When I got home this evening—hours after my parents had brought Maeve home and put her to bed—I walked through the kitchen picking up fresh dog turds that Calvin had laid down like Hansel and Gretel's breadcrumbs.

 I didn't know what to do with myself, and so I finally went outside, got the snow shovel, and stepped gingerly onto the rink. There was a crack, like what you hear when you run an ice-cube tray under the tap. But then there was silence, and no movement. I stood with my full weight on the ice, and nothing moved. I shoveled, back and forth, back and forth, and then I went inside and put on my skates. I went back out, got a stick and a puck, and began skating. I glided slowly at first, waiting for my skate blades to hit a crevice and split it open. But the ice was solid, smooth. I pushed off harder, twisted around and skated backwards, began flipping the puck against a piece of plywood I've mounted at one end. Then I began hitting slapshots, the thwack and the boom echoing through the neighborhood. People are going to be pissed, I thought, but I hit some more.

 I skated hard for an hour, and I felt as if I were flying, as Maeve said of herself when she had that fever in December. It was silent, except for the cut of my skate blades in the ice, the thwack of the puck. Eventually, it began snowing lightly, and after a little while there was just the thinnest layer on the ice, so that the puck made tracks in it.

 After I finally quit, exhausted, I went to bed sweaty, my heart pounding.

 And when I got up twice more in the night to take the dog out, carrying him down the slippery steps, I stepped out onto the ice again, and I stood there shivering, while Calvin peed and obsessively ate snow. Maura, I imagined, was awake at the same moments, breastfeeding the baby.

JANUARY 17

Saturday. It wasn't just the turds on the kitchen floor, or the trips out into the cold night, or even the shit I cleaned up this morning from the place where Calvin slept at the foot of the bed. Or maybe it *was* all of that, piled on to the exhausting confusion and doubts of the last two weeks, and combined with some sense of freedom or responsibility that hit me during the night—the need or chance to get important things in order while Maura is consumed with her own business. However it all added up, this morning seemed the right time to end the misery and uncertainty and anxiety in this other realm of our lives. And in Calvin's life. I called the vet. They could fit us in at 11:20.

Maeve was going to a morning symphony concert with Curtis and his mother. I didn't tell her about Calvin before she left, deciding instead to save the news and explanation for when we were in Fergus's presence, to let him serve as distraction, as counterbalance, expiation. Not that she needs any explanation. She's witnessed the dog's decline as vividly as we have, and we've talked with her about what's likely to happen. Perry's death, the miscarriages, Gail's death—they've all paved the way for her understanding of this particular inevitability. So she would go hear some uplifting Mozart, and I'd meet her at the hospital later.

My parents spoke their own goodbyes to Calvin and scratched him behind the ears, and his enjoyment of that affection made me feel even crummier about then having to carry him out to the car. And it had to be a sunny day, the fresh snow brilliant white, the ice of the rink sparkling, the temperature almost balmy at twenty-five. Calvin stood again through the whole drive—taking in, I hope, clear views of the very kind of winter day that he has always loved, the kind during which he would nap on a snowbank for hours.

The receptionist remembered us from last week, and she cooed over Calvin for several minutes, sad to see us return. Then she sent us into the exam room. It was a pink room, cleared of everything except a blue-and-yellow-striped blanket on the floor. After Calvin had trudged over it a few times in his clockwise fashion, I saw by the tag on the underside that it was a blanket from British Airways, the thin and medium-sized kind they give you so you can sleep uncomfortably on their planes. It seemed appropriate—the flying away, the fact that Gail had been such a traveler, had likely used a blanket just like this when she flew to London on her last trip.

We waited. The room was warm, as if they'd turned up the heat for his comfort. The assistant stuck her head in once and said the doctor would be in soon, but we waited and waited. I kept feeding Calvin doggie snacks from the jar on the shelf. He must've eaten twenty of them. It kept him occupied. And I was trying to keep myself occupied, focused on the import of the moment. I tried not to think as much as I was about the baby, about Maura.

Calvin and I had time to talk. I told him what a good dog he'd been, how happy we were to have been able to have him live with us for five months, how lucky he was to be going where he and Gail could take walks together again. I whispered to him that I loved him, that Maura loved him, that Maeve loved him dearly, and that Fergus would love him if he could. I shoveled the snacks into him. They kept him standing next to me, rather than pacing in circles.

The doctor and the assistant finally arrived. It was a busy morning. The doctor had been with a woman who, for the fifth time in two weeks, had brought her cat to be euthanized. Each time she'd changed her mind—an exam-room reprieve for the suffering animal. This morning she'd finally followed through. The doctor had spent time calming her.

A string of deaths. I really didn't want to be in the midst of it.

The doctor explained what would happen. Her tone was sincere and unpracticed. I liked her immensely. Then the assistant held Calvin firmly but gently around the shoulders. I began to scratch his ribs from behind.

The needle was big and filled with pink liquid. The vet shaved a patch from his left front leg and put the needle in a vein. "Okay, the needle's in the vein and I'm going to begin to inject the medicine now," she said, giving me, as she no doubt had the cat owner, a chance to change my mind. I nodded, and she eased in the plunger. The liquid seemed viscous, the pushing slow. Calvin began to struggle a little, and then I heard his breathing get labored. He gave a few wheezes, as if a belt were tightening around his lungs. It was the sound I've heard in too-graphic movies, when someone gets shot in the neck. Everyone was talking gently to him: "That's a good boy. Yes, go ahead and relax. You're such a good dog." It took thirty seconds, maybe, before he began to collapse, to fall sideways. The assistant and I eased him to the blanket. He kept wheezing a few more times, and I saw that his lips were drawn in around his long nose, as if he'd lost his teeth. He looked years older. We all let go of him. He lay still.

"Now I'm going to check to see that the heart has stopped," said the vet. She put her stethoscope on three or four places around Calvin's chest, and then said, "Okay, the heart has stopped." We both let a few seconds of silence go by. The assistant had left the room quietly. "That's the end of an era," said the vet.

And then we stood up and talked for a few minutes about dogs to come—bigger ones and ones just as beautiful: Newfoundlands, sheepdogs, maybe another collie.

And I left Calvin lying on the blanket that was taking him on his flight. My own flight was to the hospital. I paid the bill to the receptionist, and drove with jumpiness to St. Joe's, annoyed at every red light, almost running a stop sign and nearly broadsiding an SUV. But I made it safely, and I hustled upstairs to the fifth floor, to find Maura and Fergus in a mellow feeding frenzy—him feeding and her mellow.

I whispered to her that I'd come from the vet, and tears welled up in her eyes, but we didn't talk about it more than that. Over lunch in the cafeteria a little later, I would tell Maeve, and she would accept it with her interesting mixture of perfectly expressed sympathy and articulate curiosity about the science of the procedure.

When Maura was done with the baby, I took him. I sat in a deep chair and held him while he slept. Now and then he would open his eyes ever so slightly, and I'd see pools the dark color of a pond in the woods. Almost uninterruptedly, though, he slept, and I held him, saying his name again and again silently to myself, thinking *son, son, son.*

sightline books
The Iowa Series in Literary Nonfiction

The Men in My Country
MARILYN ABILDSKOV

Shadow Girl: A Memoir of Attachment
DEB ABRAMSON

Embalming Mom: Essays in Life
JANET BURROWAY

Family Bible
MELISSA J. DELBRIDGE

Dream Not of Other Worlds: Teaching in a Segregated Elementary School, 1970
HUSTON DIEHL

Fauna and Flora, Earth and Sky: Brushes with Nature's Wisdom
TRUDY DITTMAR

In Defense of Nature
JOHN HAY

Letters to Kate: Life after Life
CARL H. KLAUS

Essays of Elia
CHARLES LAMB

The Body of Brooklyn
DAVID LAZAR

No Such Country: Essays toward Home
ELMAR LUETH

Grammar Lessons: Translating a Life in Spain
MICHELE MORANO

Currency of the Heart: A Year of Investing, Death, Work, and Coins
DONALD R. NICHOLS

Return to Warden's Grove: Science, Desire, and the Lives of Sparrows
CHRISTOPHER NORMENT

Oppenheimer Is Watching Me: A Memoir
JEFF PORTER

Great Expectation: A Father's Diary
DAN ROCHE

Memoirs of a Revolutionary
VICTOR SERGE

The Harvard Black Rock Forest
GEORGE W. S. TROW